THE COMPLETE
CKD DIET
COOKBOOK

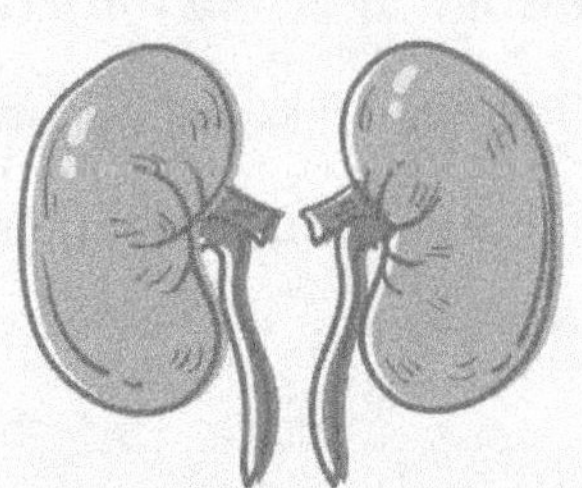

Healthy and Easy-to-Follow Low Sodium, Low Potassium, And Low Phosphorus Recipes With Expert Insights For managing Chronic Kidney Disease

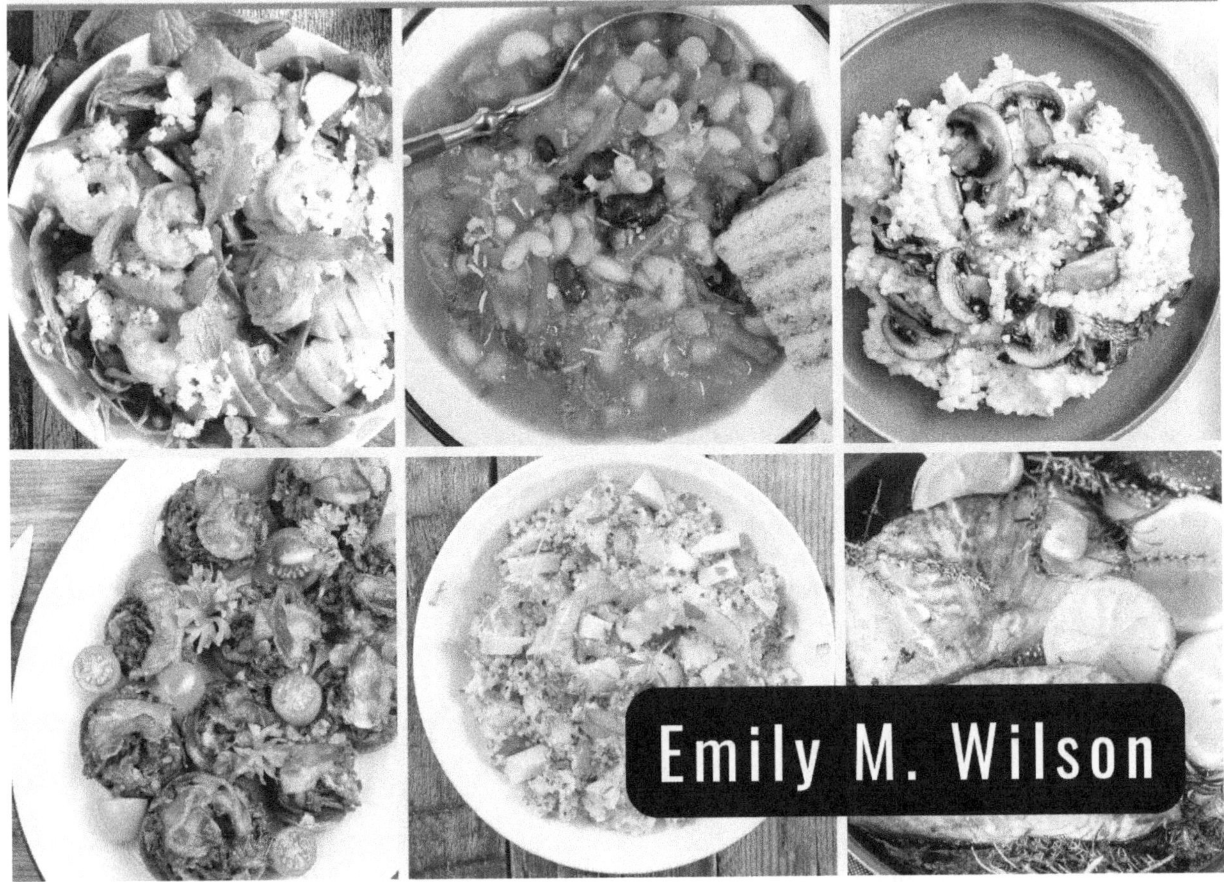

Emily M. Wilson

CONTENTS

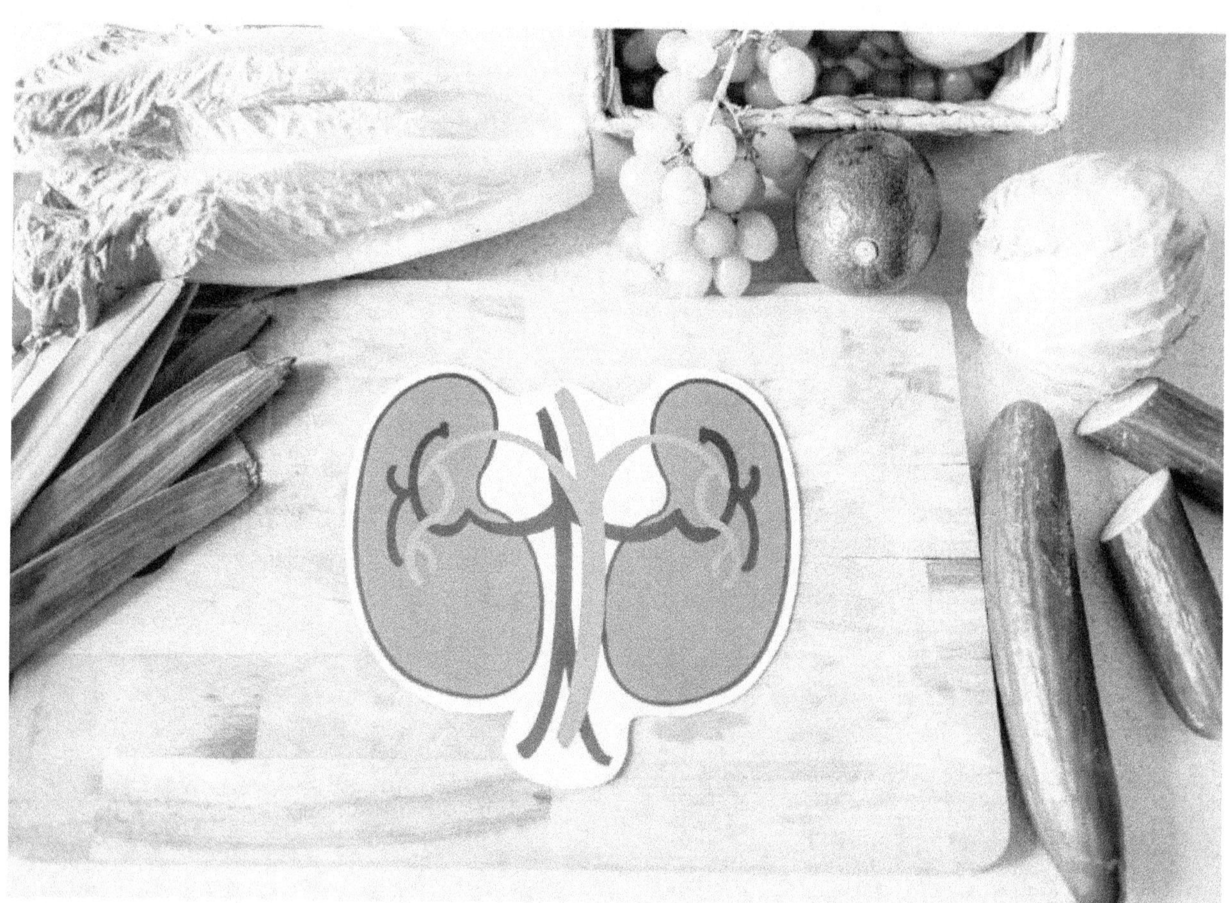

INTRODUCTION

In the bustling rhythm of modern life, health often takes a backseat to the demands of our daily routines. The realization that our well-being is intricately woven into the fabric of our habits struck me one day, a realization that eventually led to the conception of this book. My name is Emily M. Wilson, and I am not just the author of this cookbook; I am someone who, like you, is on a journey towards better health.

The seeds of this project were planted during a moment of reflection on personal health choices. As someone deeply connected to the healthcare field, I realized the gap in accessible and practical resources for those navigating the nuances of chronic conditions. It was in this space of contemplation that the idea for the "CKD Diet Cookbook" took root.

My professional journey has granted me the privilege of working closely with individuals managing various health challenges. It became evident that there was a need for a comprehensive guide tailored to those grappling with Chronic Kidney Disease. Thus, this book was born, not just as a compilation of recipes, but as a companion on your path to nourishing your kidneys and embracing a healthier lifestyle.

While the intricacies of CKD have been demystified in Chapter One, the journey is not just about understanding a medical condition; it's about empowering you to make tangible, positive changes. The recipes within these pages are a culmination of careful research, a deep understanding of nutrition, and a passion for creating meals that are not only kidney-friendly but also delicious and satisfying.

As you explore the chapters, you will find not only a diverse array of recipes but also practical insights into dietary guidelines, nutrient-rich options, and lifestyle changes that contribute to improved kidney health. Each page is a testament to the belief that nourishing our bodies can be a joyful experience, even when managing health challenges.

To make the most of this cookbook, consider it as more than a collection of recipes; think of it as a tool to reframe the way you approach food. Whether you are embarking on a 30-day meal plan or incorporating individual recipes into your routine, this book is designed to be a flexible and empowering resource. It's about making choices that resonate with your health goals and align with your taste preferences.

Remember, this journey is yours to navigate, and this book is here to guide you. The power to embrace a healthier, kidney-friendly lifestyle is within your reach. Through mindful choices and a commitment to your well-being, you are not just managing a condition; you are fostering a foundation for a vibrant and wholesome life.

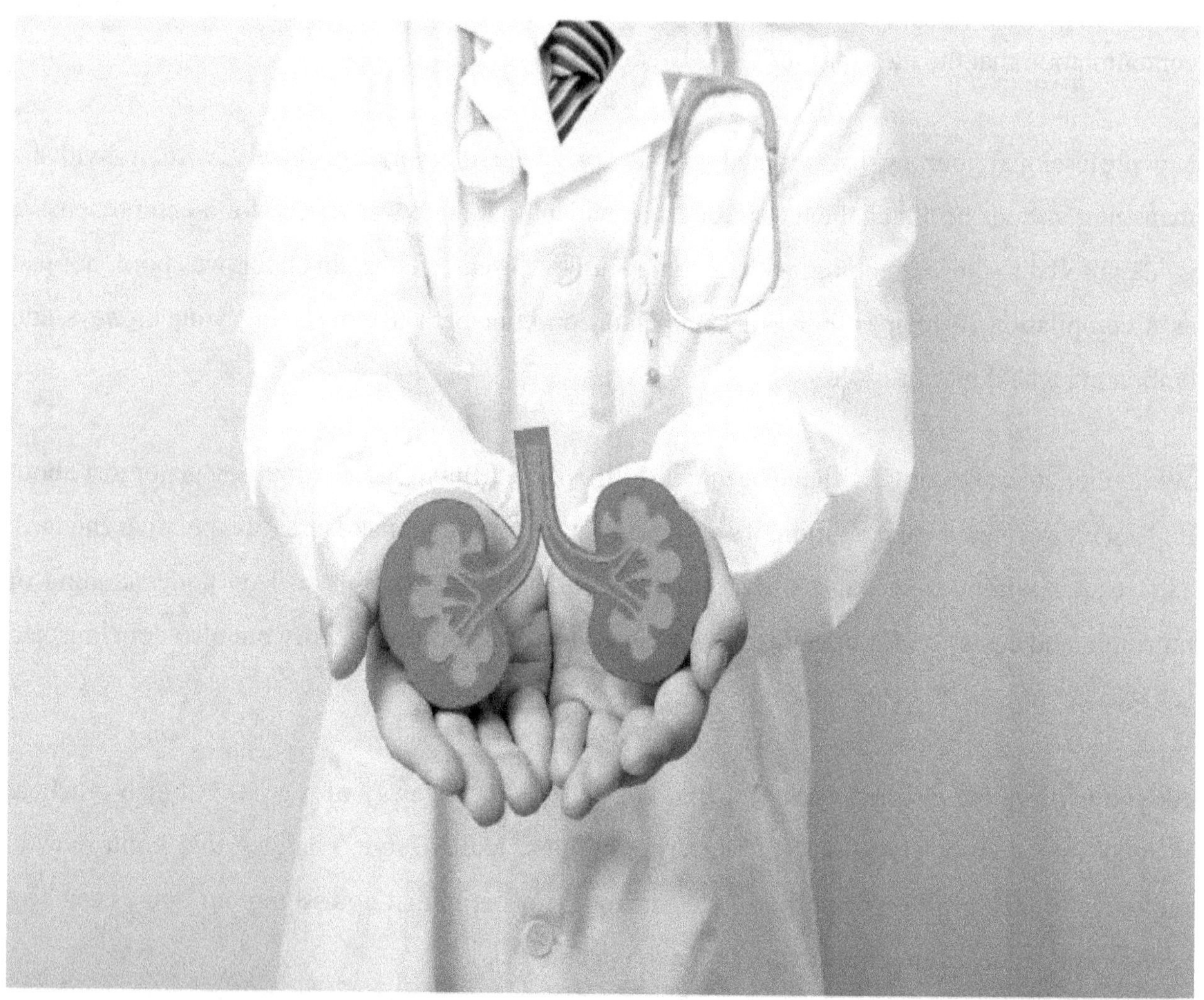

CHAPTER ONE: UNDERSTANDING CHRONIC KIDNEY DISEASE

WHAT IS CHRONIC KIDNEY DISEASE (CKD) AND ITS IMPLICATIONS?

Chronic Kidney Disease (CKD) is a complex and debilitating medical condition that warrants thorough understanding and attention due to its profound impact on an individual's health and quality of life. It is characterized by the gradual and often irreversible loss of kidney function over an extended period.

Unlike Acute Kidney Injury (AKI), which can result from sudden trauma, infections, or medication toxicity and is potentially reversible with prompt treatment, CKD is a chronic, progressive condition. This means that CKD develops over months or years, slowly affecting the kidneys' ability to perform their vital functions effectively.

The implications of CKD are multifaceted and extend beyond the kidneys themselves. Here are some key points to consider:

- **Systemic Impact:** CKD is not confined to the kidneys alone; it has far-reaching effects on various organ systems in the body. As kidney function declines, the accumulation of waste products, electrolyte imbalances, and fluid retention can have detrimental effects on other vital organs, such as the heart, brain, and lungs.

- **Cardiovascular Risk:** CKD significantly elevates the risk of cardiovascular disease, including heart attacks and strokes. The kidneys play a crucial role in regulating blood pressure and maintaining fluid balance. When they malfunction, blood pressure can become difficult to control, leading to damage to the heart and blood vessels.

- **Anemia:** The kidneys produce erythropoietin, a hormone that stimulates the production of red blood cells in the bone marrow. In CKD, the reduced production of erythropoietin can result in anemia, leading to fatigue, weakness, and decreased oxygen-carrying capacity in the blood.

- **Bone Health:** CKD can disrupt the balance of calcium and phosphorus in the body, affecting bone health. This imbalance can lead to conditions like renal osteodystrophy, causing bone pain, fractures, and deformities.
- **Electrolyte Imbalances:** Kidneys regulate the levels of electrolytes such as sodium, potassium, and calcium in the blood. In CKD, electrolyte imbalances can arise, potentially causing muscle cramps, irregular heart rhythms, and other complications.
- **Nutritional Challenges:** As CKD progresses, dietary restrictions may be necessary to manage electrolyte imbalances and reduce the burden on the kidneys. This can be challenging for individuals, impacting their quality of life and nutritional status.
- **Psychological and Emotional Impact:** Coping with a chronic condition like CKD can take a toll on an individual's mental and emotional well-being. The need for ongoing medical appointments, dietary restrictions, and concerns about disease progression can lead to anxiety and depression.
- **Quality of Life:** CKD can ultimately progress to end-stage kidney disease (ESKD), where the kidneys are no longer able to perform their essential functions. At this stage, individuals may require kidney replacement therapy, such as dialysis or kidney transplantation, which can significantly impact their lifestyle and daily activities.

Given the far-reaching implications of CKD on an individual's health, it is crucial for healthcare professionals and patients alike to be proactive in its management. Early diagnosis, lifestyle modifications, and appropriate medical interventions can help slow the progression of CKD and mitigate its effects. Additionally, raising awareness and understanding of CKD among the general population is essential to promote early detection and improve outcomes for those affected by this chronic condition.

STAGES OF CKD

Chronic Kidney Disease (CKD) is categorized into _five distinct stages,_ each representing a different level of kidney function. These stages are crucial for healthcare professionals to assess the severity of the disease, determine appropriate treatments, and predict potential outcomes. The stages are as follows:

Stage 1: Kidney damage with normal or high glomerular filtration rate (GFR)

In this stage, kidney function remains relatively normal, but there may be evidence of kidney damage, such as the presence of protein in the urine or abnormal imaging findings. The GFR is equal to or greater than 90 mL/min.

Stage 2: Mild reduction in GFR

Here, there is a slight decline in kidney function, but it is still relatively mild. GFR ranges from 60 to 89 mL/min. People at this stage may not exhibit noticeable symptoms, but medical monitoring is essential to manage any underlying conditions contributing to CKD.

Stage 3: Moderate reduction in GFR

Stage 3 CKD is divided into two sub-stages:

- **Stage 3A: GFR between 45 and 59 mL/min**
- **Stage 3B: GFR between 30 and 44 mL/min**

At this point, individuals may start to experience symptoms like fatigue, fluid retention, and changes in urination patterns. Medical intervention becomes more critical to slow the progression of CKD and address associated complications.

Stage 4: Severe reduction in GFR

Stage 4 CKD is characterized by a significant decrease in kidney function, with GFR ranging from 15 to 29 mL/min. Symptoms become more pronounced, and individuals often experience complications such as anemia, bone disease, and electrolyte imbalances. Preparations for kidney replacement therapy may begin at this stage.

Stage 5: End-stage kidney disease (ESKD) with very low GFR

In this final stage, kidney function is severely compromised, with a GFR of less than 15 mL/min. ESKD necessitates kidney replacement therapy, either through dialysis or kidney transplantation, to maintain life. Without intervention, the accumulation of waste products and fluid imbalance can become life-threatening.

COMMON CAUSES OF CKD

Understanding the underlying causes of CKD is vital for prevention and early intervention. Several factors contribute to the development of CKD:

1. **Diabetes:** Uncontrolled diabetes is one of the leading causes of CKD. High blood sugar levels can damage the small blood vessels in the kidneys over time, impairing their function.
2. **Hypertension (High Blood Pressure):** Persistent high blood pressure can strain the delicate blood vessels in the kidneys, leading to kidney damage.
3. **Glomerulonephritis:** Inflammation of the glomeruli, the tiny filtering units in the kidneys, can result from infections, autoimmune disorders, or other conditions, contributing to CKD.
4. **Polycystic Kidney Disease:** A genetic disorder characterized by the growth of fluid-filled cysts in the kidneys, which can lead to kidney damage over time.
5. **Autoimmune Diseases:** Conditions such as lupus and vasculitis can affect the kidneys and cause inflammation and damage.
6. **Urinary Tract Obstructions:** Blockages in the urinary tract, such as kidney stones or tumors, can impair kidney function and lead to CKD.

Medications and Toxins: Certain medications and environmental toxins can harm the kidneys if used or encountered inappropriately.

KIDNEY FUNCTION AND ITS IMPORTANCE

The kidneys are remarkable organs with several vital functions in the body:

Filtration: Their primary role is to filter waste products and excess fluids from the bloodstream, creating urine for elimination.

Fluid Balance: Kidneys help regulate the balance of fluids and electrolytes (sodium, potassium, calcium) in the body, maintaining proper hydration and blood pressure.

Blood Pressure Regulation: They play a crucial role in controlling blood pressure through the renin-angiotensin-aldosterone system, adjusting blood vessel diameter and fluid volume.

Red Blood Cell Production: The kidneys produce erythropoietin, a hormone that stimulates the bone marrow to create red blood cells, ensuring adequate oxygen transport in the bloodstream..

DIAGNOSING CHRONIC KIDNEY DISEASE

Early diagnosis of CKD is essential for timely intervention. Diagnosing CKD involves a systematic approach:

Medical History: Healthcare professionals take a detailed medical history, including risk factors like diabetes, hypertension, family history of kidney disease, and medication use.

Physical Examination: A physical exam may reveal signs of kidney disease, such as fluid retention, high blood pressure, or abnormal abdominal masses.

Laboratory Tests: Key laboratory tests include:

- **Serum Creatinine:** A blood test that measures waste product levels. Elevated creatinine levels indicate reduced kidney function.
- **Estimated Glomerular Filtration Rate (eGFR):** Calculated based on creatinine levels, eGFR estimates how efficiently the kidneys filter blood. A lower eGFR indicates reduced kidney function.
- **Urinary Albumin-to-Creatinine Ratio (UACR):** A urine test that assesses the amount of protein (albumin) in the urine. Elevated UACR may signify kidney damage.
- **Imaging Studies:** Imaging tests like ultrasound or CT scans may be used to visualize the kidneys and detect structural abnormalities.

KIDNEY FUNCTION NUMBERS

Here's a simplified tabular representation of key kidney function numbers and their significance:

Indicator	Normal Range	Significance in CKD
Serum Creatinine	Varies by age and gender	Elevated levels indicate reduced kidney function
Estimated GFR (eGFR)	≥ 90 mL/min (Stage 1)	Decreasing eGFR values indicate CKD progression
Urinary Albumin-to-Creatinine Ratio (UACR)	< 30 mg/g (normal)	Elevated UACR suggests kidney damage

Understanding these numbers helps individuals and healthcare providers monitor kidney health and make informed decisions regarding CKD management, including lifestyle changes and medical interventions.

Comprehending the impact of CKD on kidney function, the diagnostic process, relevant tests and indicators, recognizing early signs, and understanding kidney function numbers are essential components of managing this chronic condition effectively. Early detection and intervention can significantly improve outcomes and enhance the quality of life for individuals living with CKD.

CHAPTER TWO: MANAGING CKD THROUGH DIET AND LIFESTYLE CHANGES

IMPORTANCE OF DIET IN CHRONIC KIDNEY DISEASE

Chronic Kidney Disease (CKD) necessitates a heightened awareness of dietary choices due to the direct impact nutrition has on kidney function. A well-managed diet plays a pivotal role in slowing the progression of CKD and mitigating associated complications. Understanding the importance of a kidney-friendly diet is foundational to the overall health and well-being of individuals grappling with CKD.

DIETARY GUIDELINES FOR CHRONIC KIDNEY DISEASE (CKD)

Managing Chronic Kidney Disease requires a strategic and thoughtful approach to diet. The following dietary guidelines are instrumental in supporting kidney health and slowing the progression of CKD:

1. Controlled Protein Intake

1. Moderation in protein consumption is crucial to alleviate the burden on the kidneys. High-protein diets can contribute to increased waste products, potentially accelerating kidney damage. Tailoring protein intake to individual needs, often under the guidance of a healthcare professional, is a key aspect of CKD dietary management.

2. Phosphorus Awareness

2. Monitoring phosphorus levels is essential for CKD patients, as impaired kidney function can lead to difficulty in eliminating excess phosphorus. Excessive phosphorus can contribute to bone and cardiovascular issues. Choosing foods with lower phosphorus content and utilizing phosphate binders, when necessary, helps maintain a healthy balance.

3. Potassium Moderation

3. As the kidneys struggle to regulate potassium levels in CKD, it becomes crucial to manage potassium intake. High potassium levels can lead to irregular heartbeats and other complications. Guided by healthcare professionals, individuals with CKD should focus on consuming foods with controlled potassium content.

4. Limited Sodium Intake

4. Sodium restriction is pivotal in managing CKD-related hypertension and fluid retention. Reducing the consumption of processed and salty foods helps maintain optimal blood pressure levels. Emphasizing fresh, whole foods and using herbs and spices for flavoring are effective strategies to lower sodium intake.

5. Fluid Control

5. Monitoring fluid intake is essential for CKD patients, particularly those experiencing fluid retention. Balancing hydration with the body's ability to eliminate excess fluids helps prevent complications such as edema and high blood pressure. Individual fluid restrictions may be recommended based on the severity of CKD.

RENAL-FRIENDLY FOODS TO INCLUDE

In crafting a renal-friendly diet, the focus is on selecting foods that provide essential nutrients without overburdening the kidneys. Here are key categories of renal-friendly foods:

1. Low-Potassium Fruits And Vegetables	Incorporating fruits like apples, berries, and vegetables such as cabbage and green beans ensures a balance of vitamins and minerals without excessive potassium.
2. Lean Proteins	Opting for lean protein sources, such as poultry, fish, and eggs, helps meet protein needs without overloading the

	kidneys. Plant-based proteins like tofu and legumes are also valuable alternatives.
3. Whole Grains	Whole grains like brown rice, quinoa, and whole wheat provide essential nutrients and fiber without contributing excessive phosphorus.
4. Healthy Fats	Choosing sources of healthy fats, such as avocados and olive oil, supports overall health without negatively impacting kidney function.
5. Calcium-Rich Foods	While phosphorus control is important, including moderate amounts of calcium-rich foods like low-fat dairy or fortified alternatives helps maintain bone health.

FOODS TO AVOID FOR KIDNEY HEALTH

Certain foods should be limited or avoided to prevent further strain on compromised kidneys. Key considerations include:

1. High-Potassium Foods	Bananas, oranges, tomatoes, and potatoes are examples of foods high in potassium that should be consumed in moderation or avoided, depending on individual needs.
2. High-Phosphorus Foods	Dairy products, nuts, seeds, and processed foods often contain elevated phosphorus levels and may need to be restricted or carefully managed.

3. Sodium-Rich Foods	Processed and canned foods, as well as high-sodium condiments, contribute to elevated sodium levels. Reducing these items supports blood pressure control and overall kidney health.
Excessive Protein Sources	Limiting red meat, processed meats, and excessive protein intake helps manage kidney workload and reduces the production of waste products.

Adherence to these dietary guidelines, with individualized adjustments based on medical advice, is integral to promoting kidney health and improving the quality of life for individuals living with CKD.

COOKING METHODS FOR KIDNEY HEALTH

Choosing kidney-friendly cooking methods is an essential aspect of maintaining a healthful diet for individuals with kidney concerns. By focusing on techniques that preserve nutrient content and minimize the use of additives detrimental to renal health, individuals can support their kidneys while still enjoying flavorful meals. Here are key considerations for kidney-friendly cooking methods:

1. Baking and Roasting

- Baking and roasting are excellent methods that enhance the natural flavors of foods without the need for excessive fats or sodium. These techniques result in delicious and nutrient-rich dishes, making them suitable for a kidney-friendly diet.

2. Grilling and Broiling

- Grilling and broiling are ideal for imparting a smoky flavor to meats and vegetables without the need for added fats. These methods are particularly effective for lean proteins, providing a satisfying culinary experience while aligning with kidney health goals.

3. Steaming

- Steaming is a gentle cooking method that helps retain the nutritional value of foods. It is particularly beneficial for vegetables and fish, ensuring that essential vitamins and minerals are preserved without the need for added fats or salt.

4. Sautéing with Minimal Oil

- Sautéing with a minimal amount of healthy oils, such as olive oil, adds flavor to dishes without compromising kidney health. This method allows for the development of rich, savory profiles without excessive saturated fats.

5. Avoiding Deep-Frying

- Deep-frying introduces unnecessary fats and calories to meals, which can be detrimental to kidney health. Opting for alternative cooking methods preserves the nutritional integrity of foods without compromising their flavor.

By incorporating these kidney-friendly cooking methods, you can create meals that are not only enjoyable but also supportive of overall renal health.

LIFESTYLE CHANGES FOR IMPROVED KIDNEY HEALTH

Beyond dietary considerations, embracing lifestyle changes is crucial for individuals looking to optimize kidney health and manage chronic kidney conditions. Here are key lifestyle changes that contribute to improved kidney health:

1. **Adequate Hydration:** Staying well-hydrated is fundamental for supporting kidney function. Sufficient water intake helps flush out toxins and waste products, reducing the risk of kidney-related complications. Individuals should aim for a balance between hydration and fluid restrictions, guided by healthcare professionals.

2. **Regular Exercise:** Engaging in regular physical activity contributes to overall health and can positively impact kidney function. Exercise helps regulate blood pressure, manage weight, and enhance cardiovascular health—important factors in maintaining optimal kidney function.

3. **Maintaining a Healthy Weight:** Achieving and maintaining a healthy weight is crucial for individuals with kidney concerns. A balanced diet, portion control, and regular exercise contribute to weight management, reducing the risk of complications associated with obesity and kidney issues.

4. **Managing Blood Pressure:** Hypertension is a common complication of kidney disease. Lifestyle changes, including dietary modifications, regular exercise, and stress management, play pivotal roles in maintaining optimal blood pressure levels. Regular monitoring and collaboration with healthcare professionals are essential.

5. **Avoiding Smoking and Excessive Alcohol Consumption:** Smoking and excessive alcohol consumption can exacerbate kidney damage. Quitting smoking and moderating alcohol intake are key lifestyle changes that positively impact overall health and contribute to kidney health.

6. **Regular Medical Check-ups:** Regular medical check-ups and consultations with healthcare professionals are essential for individuals with kidney concerns. Monitoring kidney function through blood tests and other diagnostic tools allows for early detection of issues and timely intervention.

Embracing these lifestyle changes, in conjunction with a kidney-friendly diet, creates a holistic approach to kidney health. Individuals are encouraged to work closely with healthcare professionals to tailor lifestyle adjustments to their specific needs and optimize overall well-being.

1. BREAKFAST

VEGETABLE OMELETTE

Prep/Cook Time: 15 minutes

Ingredients (for one serving):

- 2 large eggs
- 1/4 cup bell peppers, diced
- 1/4 cup tomatoes, diced
- 1/4 cup spinach, chopped
- Salt and pepper to taste

Cooking Instructions:

1. Whisk eggs in a bowl and season with salt and pepper.
2. In a non-stick pan, sauté bell peppers, tomatoes, and spinach until softened.
3. Pour the whisked eggs over the veggies and cook until the edges set.
4. Fold the omelette in half and cook until eggs are fully cooked.

Nutritional Information:

- Calories: 250
- Protein: 18g
- Carbohydrates: 7g
- Fat: 16g
- Fiber: 2g

- Add low-phosphorus cheese for extra flavor.
- Incorporate fresh herbs like parsley or chives for added freshness.

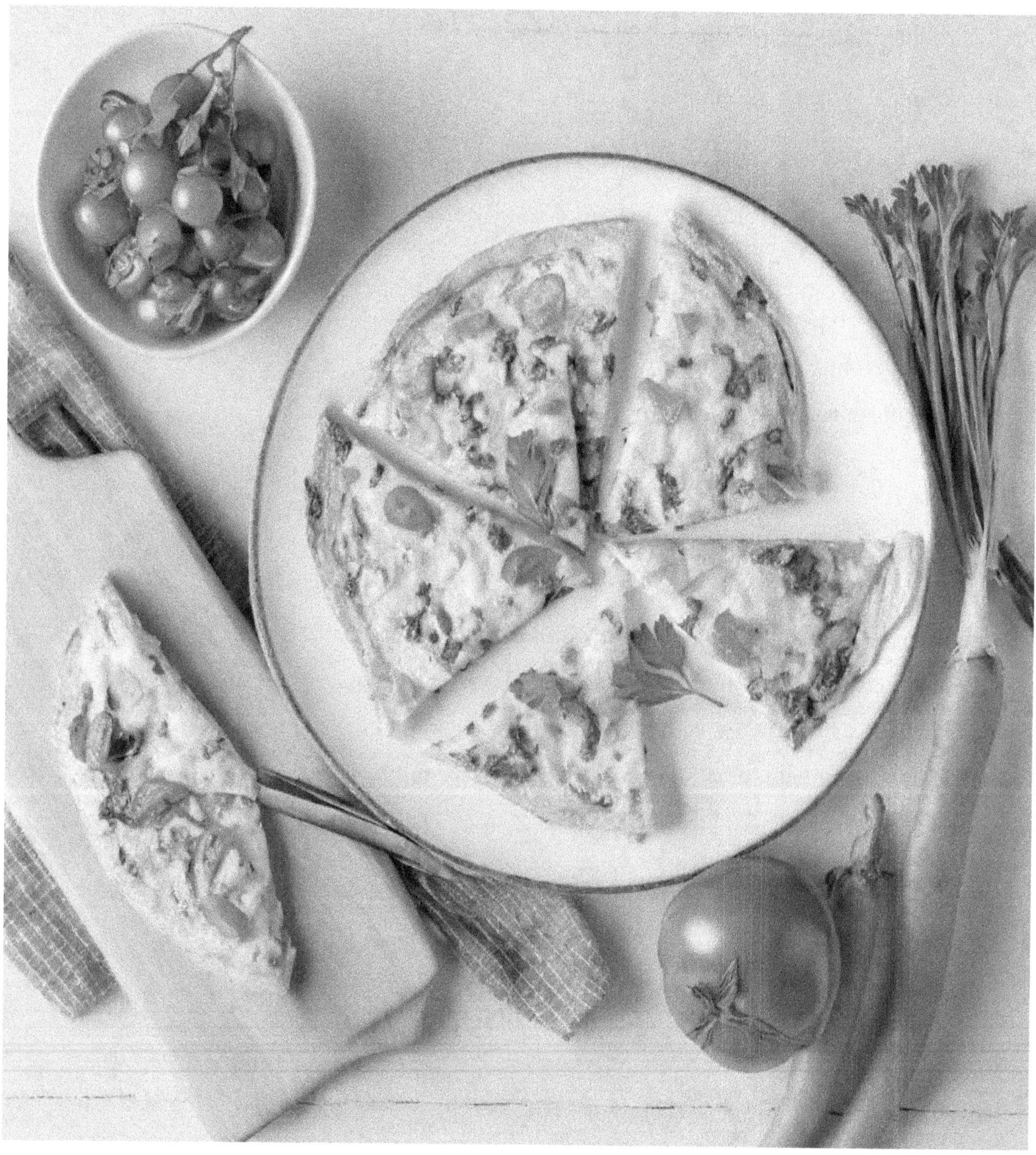

QUINOA BREAKFAST BOWL

Prep/Cook Time: 20 minutes

Ingredients (for one serving):

- 1/2 cup cooked quinoa
- 1/4 cup berries (blueberries, strawberries)
- 1 tablespoon chopped nuts (almonds, walnuts)
- 1 teaspoon honey
- 1/4 cup low-fat yogurt

Cooking Instructions:

1. Cook quinoa according to package instructions.
2. In a bowl, combine quinoa, berries, nuts, and honey.
3. Top with a dollop of low-fat yogurt.

Nutritional Information:

- Calories: 300
- Protein: 8g
- Carbohydrates: 45g
- Fat: 10g
- Fiber: 5g

Tips for Recipe Modification:

- Use a sugar substitute instead of honey for a lower-sugar option.
- Add a sprinkle of cinnamon for extra flavor.

SWEET POTATO HASH

Prep/Cook Time: 25 minutes

Ingredients (for one serving):

- 1/2 cup sweet potatoes, diced
- 1/4 cup onions, chopped
- 1/4 cup bell peppers, diced
- 1 tablespoon olive oil
- Salt and pepper to taste

Cooking Instructions:

1. In a skillet, heat olive oil over medium heat.
2. Add sweet potatoes, onions, and bell peppers. Cook until sweet potatoes are tender.
3. Season with salt and pepper to taste.

Nutritional Information:

- Calories: 220
- Protein: 2g
- Carbohydrates: 30g
- Fat: 11g
- Fiber: 4g

Tips for Recipe Modification:

- Add kidney-friendly herbs like thyme or rosemary.
- Serve with a poached egg for extra protein.

Prep/Cook Time: 10 minutes

Ingredients (for one serving):

- 1/2 cup low-fat Greek yogurt
- 1/4 cup granola (low-phosphorus)
- 1/4 cup fresh berries
- 1 teaspoon honey

Cooking Instructions:

1. In a glass, layer Greek yogurt, granola, and fresh berries.
2. Drizzle honey over the top.

Nutritional Information:

- Calories: 250
- Protein: 15g
- Carbohydrates: 35g
- Fat: 6g
- Fiber: 4g

Tips for Recipe Modification:

- Choose a granola with lower phosphorus content.
- Add chopped nuts for extra crunch.

Prep/Cook Time: 15 minutes

Ingredients (for one serving):

- 1/2 cup low-fat cottage cheese
- 2 tablespoons oat flour
- 1 large egg
- 1/2 teaspoon baking powder
- 1/4 teaspoon vanilla extract

Cooking Instructions:

1. In a bowl, mix cottage cheese, oat flour, egg, baking powder, and vanilla extract.
2. Heat a non-stick pan and spoon batter to form pancakes.
3. Cook until bubbles form, then flip and cook until golden brown.

Nutritional Information:

- Calories: 280
- Protein: 25g
- Carbohydrates: 20g
- Fat: 10g
- Fiber: 2g

Tips for Recipe Modification:

- Serve with fresh fruit instead of syrup.
- Add a dash of cinnamon for extra flavor.

EGG AND SPINACH BREAKFAST WRAP

Prep/Cook Time: 15 minutes

Ingredients (for one serving):

- 1 whole-grain tortilla
- 2 large eggs, scrambled
- 1/2 cup spinach, sautéed
- 1/4 cup feta cheese, crumbled

Cooking Instructions:

1. In a pan, scramble eggs until cooked.
2. Sauté spinach until wilted.
3. Place eggs and spinach on a tortilla, top with feta, and fold.

Nutritional Information:

- Calories: 320
- Protein: 20g
- Carbohydrates: 25g
- Fat: 15g
- Fiber: 5g

Tips for Recipe Modification:

- Use a whole-grain or low-carb tortilla.
- Add diced tomatoes for freshness.

Prep/Cook Time: 8 hours (overnight soaking)

Ingredients (for one serving):

- 2 tablespoons chia seeds
- 1/2 cup unsweetened almond milk
- 1/4 teaspoon vanilla extract
- 1/2 tablespoon maple syrup
- 1/4 cup fresh berries

Cooking Instructions:

1. Mix chia seeds, almond milk, vanilla extract, and maple syrup in a jar.
2. Refrigerate overnight.
3. Top with fresh berries before serving.

Nutritional Information:

- Calories: 180
- Protein: 5g
- Carbohydrates: 25g
- Fat: 8g
- Fiber: 10g

Tips for Recipe Modification:

- Experiment with different non-dairy milk options.
- Add a sprinkle of chopped nuts for texture.

Prep/Cook Time: 20 minutes

Ingredients (for one serving):

- 2 large eggs
- 1/2 cup mushrooms, sliced
- 1/2 cup spinach, chopped
- 1/4 cup feta cheese, crumbled
- Salt and pepper to taste

Cooking Instructions:

1. Whisk eggs in a bowl and season with salt and pepper.
2. In an oven-safe pan, sauté mushrooms and spinach until wilted.
3. Pour whisked eggs over the vegetables, top with feta, and bake until set.

Nutritional Information:

- Calories: 280
- Protein: 20g
- Carbohydrates: 6g
- Fat: 20g
- Fiber: 2g

Tips for Recipe Modification:

- Add diced bell peppers for extra color.
- Substitute goat cheese for feta for a different flavor.

Prep/Cook Time: 20 minutes

Ingredients (for one serving):

- 1/2 cup almond flour
- 1/4 teaspoon baking powder
- 2 large eggs
- 1/4 cup unsweetened almond milk
- 1/2 teaspoon vanilla extract

Cooking Instructions:

1. In a bowl, mix almond flour, baking powder, eggs, almond milk, and vanilla extract.
2. Heat a non-stick pan and spoon batter to form pancakes.
3. Cook until bubbles form, then flip and cook until golden brown.

Nutritional Information:

- Calories: 320
- Protein: 14g
- Carbohydrates: 8g
- Fat: 27g
- Fiber: 4g

Tips for Recipe Modification:

- Top with fresh berries instead of syrup.
- Add a sprinkle of cinnamon for extra flavor.

TOMATO AND BASIL EGG MUFFINS

Prep/Cook Time: 25 minutes

Ingredients (for one serving):

- 2 large eggs
- 1/4 cup cherry tomatoes, halved
- 1 tablespoon fresh basil, chopped
- Salt and pepper to taste

Cooking Instructions:

1. Preheat the oven to 350°F (175°C).
2. In a bowl, whisk eggs and season with salt and pepper.
3. Grease muffin tin cups and pour the egg mixture.
4. Add cherry tomatoes and basil on top.
5. Bake for 15-18 minutes or until eggs are set.

Nutritional Information:

- Calories: 180
- Protein: 12g
- Carbohydrates: 4g
- Fat: 13g
- Fiber: 1g

Tips for Recipe Modification:

- Incorporate low-phosphorus cheese if desired.
- Add a pinch of garlic powder for extra flavor.

PEANUT BUTTER BANANA SMOOTHIE

Prep/Cook Time: 5 minutes

Ingredients (for one serving):

- 1/2 banana, frozen
- 1 tablespoon peanut butter
- 1/2 cup unsweetened almond milk
- 1/4 teaspoon cinnamon
- Ice cubes (optional)

Cooking Instructions:

1. Blend banana, peanut butter, almond milk, and cinnamon until smooth.
2. Add ice cubes if a colder consistency is desired.

Nutritional Information:

- Calories: 250
- Protein: 8g
- Carbohydrates: 20g
- Fat: 16g
- Fiber: 4g

Tips for Recipe Modification:

- Use a sugar substitute for a lower-sugar option.
- Add a scoop of protein powder for extra protein.

SPINACH AND TOMATO BREAKFAST WRAP

Prep/Cook Time: 15 minutes

Ingredients (for one serving):

- 1 whole-grain tortilla
- 1/2 cup fresh spinach
- 1/4 cup cherry tomatoes, sliced
- 1 tablespoon feta cheese, crumbled
- 1 large egg, scrambled

Cooking Instructions:

1. In a pan, scramble the egg until cooked.
2. Heat the tortilla and place spinach, tomatoes, scrambled egg, and feta in the center.
3. Fold the sides and roll to create a wrap.

Nutritional Information:

- Calories: 280
- Protein: 14g
- Carbohydrates: 25g
- Fat: 15g
- Fiber: 4g

Tips for Recipe Modification:

- Use a low-carb or gluten-free tortilla if needed.
- Add a dash of hot sauce for a spicy kick.

BLUEBERRY ALMOND MUFFINS

Prep/Cook Time: 25 minutes

Ingredients (for one serving):

- 1/2 cup almond flour
- 1/4 teaspoon baking powder
- 1 large egg
- 1/4 cup unsweetened almond milk
- 1/4 cup blueberries

Cooking Instructions:

1. Preheat the oven to 350°F (175°C).
2. In a bowl, mix almond flour, baking powder, egg, and almond milk.
3. Gently fold in the blueberries.
4. Spoon the batter into muffin cups and bake for 18-20 minutes.

Nutritional Information:

- Calories: 280
- Protein: 10g
- Carbohydrates: 10g
- Fat: 23g
- Fiber: 4g

Tips for Recipe Modification:

- Add a touch of almond extract for extra flavor.
- Use a sugar substitute for a lower-sugar option.

CINNAMON RAISIN OVERNIGHT OATS

Prep/Cook Time: 5 minutes (plus overnight soaking)

Ingredients (for one serving):

- 1/2 cup old-fashioned oats
- 1/2 cup unsweetened almond milk
- 1/4 teaspoon cinnamon
- 1 tablespoon raisins
- 1 teaspoon honey

Cooking Instructions:

1. In a jar, combine oats, almond milk, cinnamon, raisins, and honey.
2. Refrigerate overnight.
3. Stir before serving and add more almond milk if desired.

Nutritional Information:

- Calories: 280
- Protein: 8g
- Carbohydrates: 45g
- Fat: 6g
- Fiber: 7g

Tips for Recipe Modification:

- Add chopped nuts for extra crunch.
- Use a sugar substitute for a lower-sugar option.

SALMON AND AVOCADO TOAST

Prep/Cook Time: 10 minutes

Ingredients (for one serving):

- 1 slice whole-grain bread
- 2 ounces smoked salmon
- 1/4 avocado, sliced
- Lemon juice
- Fresh dill for garnish

Cooking Instructions:

1. Toast the bread to your liking.
2. Layer sliced avocado on the toast.
3. Top with smoked salmon, a squeeze of lemon juice, and fresh dill.

Nutritional Information:

- Calories: 300
- Protein: 15g
- Carbohydrates: 25g
- Fat: 15g
- Fiber: 5g

Tips for Recipe Modification:

- Add a poached egg for extra protein.
- Sprinkle with capers for a burst of flavor.

GRILLED LEMON HERB CHICKEN

Prep/Cook Time: 30 minutes

Ingredients (for one serving):

- 4 ounces chicken breast
- 1 tablespoon olive oil
- 1 teaspoon lemon zest
- 1 teaspoon fresh herbs (rosemary, thyme)
- Salt and pepper to taste

Cooking Instructions:

1. Marinate chicken in olive oil, lemon zest, herbs, salt, and pepper.
2. Grill until fully cooked, approximately 15 minutes per side.

Nutritional Information:

- Calories: 250
- Protein: 30g
- Carbohydrates: 0g
- Fat: 14g
- Fiber: 0g

Tips for Recipe Modification:

- Serve with a side of steamed vegetables.
- Use a low-sodium herb blend to reduce salt intake.

QUINOA SALAD WITH VEGETABLES

Prep/Cook Time: 20 minutes

Ingredients (for one serving):

- 1/2 cup cooked quinoa
- 1/4 cup cucumber, diced
- 1/4 cup cherry tomatoes, halved
- 2 tablespoons red onion, finely chopped
- 1 tablespoon olive oil
- Fresh lemon juice

Cooking Instructions:

1. Combine quinoa, cucumber, tomatoes, and red onion in a bowl.
2. Drizzle with olive oil and lemon juice. Toss to combine.

Nutritional Information:

- Calories: 280
- Protein: 8g
- Carbohydrates: 40g
- Fat: 10g
- Fiber: 6g

Tips for Recipe Modification:

- Add feta cheese for extra flavor.
- Include fresh herbs like parsley or mint.

BAKED SALMON WITH ASPARAGUS

Prep/Cook Time: 25 minutes

Ingredients (for one serving):

- 4 ounces salmon fillet
- 1/2 bunch asparagus, trimmed
- 1 tablespoon olive oil
- Lemon slices
- Salt and pepper to taste

Cooking Instructions:

1. Preheat the oven to 375°F (190°C).
2. Place salmon and asparagus on a baking sheet.
3. Drizzle with olive oil, season with salt and pepper, and top with lemon slices.
4. Bake for 15-18 minutes or until salmon flakes easily.

Nutritional Information:

- Calories: 300
- Protein: 25g
- Carbohydrates: 8g
- Fat: 18g
- Fiber: 4g

Tips for Recipe Modification:

- Substitute asparagus with green beans or zucchini.
- Sprinkle with chopped dill for added freshness.

MEDITERRANEAN CHICKPEA SALAD

Prep/Cook Time: 15 minutes

Ingredients (for one serving):

- 1 cup canned chickpeas, drained and rinsed
- 1/4 cup cherry tomatoes, halved
- 2 tablespoons red onion, finely chopped
- 1/4 cup cucumber, diced
- 1/4 cup feta cheese, crumbled
- 1 tablespoon olive oil
- Fresh lemon juice

Cooking Instructions:

- In a bowl, combine chickpeas, tomatoes, red onion, cucumber, and feta.
- Drizzle with olive oil and lemon juice. Toss to combine.

Nutritional Information:

- Calories: 320
- Protein: 15g
- Carbohydrates: 30g
- Fat: 18g
- Fiber: 8g

Tips for Recipe Modification:

- Add olives for a Mediterranean twist.
- Include chopped parsley for extra freshness.

Prep/Cook Time: 15 minutes

Ingredients (for one serving):

- 4 ounces turkey breast, sliced
- 1 whole-grain or low-carb wrap
- 1/4 avocado, sliced
- 1 tablespoon Greek yogurt
- Lettuce and tomato slices

Cooking Instructions:

- Lay out the wrap and layer with turkey, avocado, Greek yogurt, lettuce, and tomato.
- Roll the wrap tightly and slice in half.

Nutritional Information:

- Calories: 320
- Protein: 30g
- Carbohydrates: 20g
- Fat: 15g
- Fiber: 8g

Tips for Recipe Modification:

- Use a gluten-free wrap if needed.
- Add a sprinkle of black pepper for extra flavor.

Prep/Cook Time: 30 minutes

Ingredients (for one serving):

- 1/2 eggplant, diced
- 1 cup cherry tomatoes, halved
- 1/4 cup red bell pepper, diced
- 1/4 cup onion, finely chopped
- 2 tablespoons olive oil
- Fresh basil for garnish

Cooking Instructions:

1. In a pan, sauté eggplant, cherry tomatoes, red bell pepper, and onion in olive oil until vegetables are tender.
2. Garnish with fresh basil before serving.

Nutritional Information:

- Calories: 280
- Protein: 5g
- Carbohydrates: 30g
- Fat: 18g
- Fiber: 10g

Tips for Recipe Modification:

- Add canned, low-sodium chickpeas for protein.
- Serve over quinoa for a complete meal.

Prep/Cook Time: 20 minutes

Ingredients (for one serving):

- 4 ounces shrimp, peeled and deveined
- 1 cup broccoli florets
- 1/2 cup snap peas
- 1 tablespoon olive oil
- 1 teaspoon lemon zest
- 1 clove garlic, minced

Cooking Instructions:

1. In a wok or skillet, heat olive oil and sauté shrimp until pink.
2. Add broccoli and snap peas, stir-frying until vegetables are tender.
3. Stir in lemon zest and minced garlic.

Nutritional Information:

- Calories: 250
- Protein: 25g
- Carbohydrates: 10g
- Fat: 14g
- Fiber: 4g

Tips for Recipe Modification:

- Serve over cauliflower rice for a low-carb option.
- Include a dash of low-sodium soy sauce for flavor.

Prep/Cook Time: 40 minutes

Ingredients (for one serving):

- 1/2 cup dry lentils, rinsed
- 1/4 cup carrots, diced
- 1/4 cup celery, diced
- 1/4 cup onion, finely chopped
- 1 clove garlic, minced
- 4 cups low-sodium vegetable broth
- 1 teaspoon olive oil

Cooking Instructions:

- In a pot, sauté onions and garlic in olive oil until softened.
- Add lentils, carrots, celery, and vegetable broth. Bring to a boil, then simmer until lentils are tender.

Nutritional Information:

- Calories: 280
- Protein: 18g
- Carbohydrates: 45g
- Fat: 4g
- Fiber: 12g

Tips for Recipe Modification:

- Add spinach or kale for extra greens.
- Season with herbs like thyme or bay leaves.

Prep/Cook Time: 25 minutes

Ingredients (for one serving):

- 4 ounces chicken breast, cubed
- 1/2 bell pepper, diced
- 1/2 zucchini, sliced
- 1 tablespoon olive oil
- 1 teaspoon dried oregano
- Salt and pepper to taste

Cooking Instructions:

1. Thread chicken, bell pepper, and zucchini onto skewers.
2. Mix olive oil, dried oregano, salt, and pepper. Brush onto skewers.
3. Grill or bake until chicken is cooked through.

Nutritional Information:

- Calories: 280
- Protein: 30g
- Carbohydrates: 10g
- Fat: 14g
- Fiber: 3g

Tips for Recipe Modification:

- Serve over a bed of quinoa or brown rice.
- Include cherry tomatoes for added color and flavor.

STUFFED BELL PEPPERS WITH TURKEY

Prep/Cook Time: 40 minutes

Ingredients (for one serving):

- 2 bell peppers, halved
- 4 ounces ground turkey
- 1/4 cup quinoa, cooked
- 1/4 cup black beans, canned and rinsed
- 1/4 cup tomato sauce
- 1 teaspoon taco seasoning

Cooking Instructions:

1. Preheat the oven to 375°F (190°C).
2. In a skillet, cook ground turkey until browned. Add cooked quinoa, black beans, tomato sauce, and taco seasoning.
3. Stuff bell peppers with the turkey mixture and bake for 25-30 minutes.

Nutritional Information:

- Calories: 320
- Protein: 25g
- Carbohydrates: 30g
- Fat: 12g
- Fiber: 7g

Tips for Recipe Modification:

- Use lean ground chicken as an alternative.
- Top with a dollop of Greek yogurt instead of sour cream.

EGG FRIED RICE WITH VEGETABLES

Prep/Cook Time: 20 minutes

Ingredients (for one serving):

- 1 cup cooked brown rice
- 1/2 cup mixed vegetables (peas, carrots, corn)
- 1 egg, beaten
- 1 tablespoon low-sodium soy sauce
- 1 teaspoon sesame oil

Cooking Instructions:

1. In a pan, stir-fry mixed vegetables until tender.
2. Push vegetables to one side and pour beaten egg into the pan, scrambling until cooked.
3. Add cooked brown rice, soy sauce, and sesame oil. Stir until well combined.

Nutritional Information:

- Calories: 300
- Protein: 12g
- Carbohydrates: 45g
- Fat: 8g
- Fiber: 6g

Tips for Recipe Modification:

- Include lean protein like diced chicken or tofu.
- Use low-sodium vegetable broth instead of soy sauce.

Prep/Cook Time: 25 minutes

Ingredients (for one serving):

- 4 ounces shrimp, peeled and deveined
- 1 cup broccoli florets
- 1/2 cup whole-grain pasta, cooked
- 1/4 cup grated Parmesan cheese
- 1/2 cup low-fat milk
- 1 clove garlic, minced

Cooking Instructions:

1. In a pan, sauté shrimp and garlic until shrimp are pink.
2. Add broccoli, cooked pasta, Parmesan cheese, and milk.
3. Stir until the cheese is melted and the sauce is creamy.

Nutritional Information:

- Calories: 350
- Protein: 25g
- Carbohydrates: 40g
- Fat: 12g
- Fiber: 6g

Tips for Recipe Modification:

- Use whole-grain or chickpea pasta for added fiber.
- Substitute milk with unsweetened almond milk for a lighter option.

CAULIFLOWER AND CHICKPEA CURRY

Prep/Cook Time: 35 minutes

Ingredients (for one serving):

- 1 cup cauliflower florets
- 1/2 cup canned chickpeas, drained and rinsed
- 1/4 cup onion, finely chopped
- 1/4 cup tomatoes, diced
- 1 tablespoon curry powder
- 1 tablespoon olive oil
- Fresh cilantro for garnish

Cooking Instructions:

1. In a pan, sauté onions in olive oil until translucent.
2. Add cauliflower, chickpeas, tomatoes, and curry powder. Cook until cauliflower is tender.
3. Garnish with fresh cilantro before serving.

Nutritional Information:

- Calories: 300
- Protein: 12g
- Carbohydrates: 40g
- Fat: 10g
- Fiber: 10g

Tips for Recipe Modification:

- Serve over quinoa or brown rice.
- Adjust curry powder to taste for preferred spice level.

Prep/Cook Time: 40 minutes

Ingredients (for one serving):

- 6 ounces chicken breast
- 1/4 cup spinach, cooked and drained
- 2 tablespoons feta cheese, crumbled
- 1 tablespoon olive oil
- 1 teaspoon lemon juice
- Salt and pepper to taste

Cooking Instructions:

1. Preheat the oven to 375°F (190°C).
2. Butterfly the chicken breast and stuff with cooked spinach and feta.
3. Drizzle with olive oil and lemon juice. Season with salt and pepper.
4. Bake for 25-30 minutes or until the chicken is cooked through.

Nutritional Information:

- Calories: 320
- Protein: 35g
- Carbohydrates: 2g
- Fat: 18g
- Fiber: 1g

Tips for Recipe Modification:

- Use low-fat feta for a lighter option.
- Serve with a side of steamed vegetables.

VEGETARIAN ZUCCHINI LASAGNA

Prep/Cook Time: 45 minutes

Ingredients (for one serving):

- 1 medium zucchini, sliced lengthwise
- 1/2 cup ricotta cheese
- 1/4 cup mozzarella cheese, shredded
- 1/4 cup tomato sauce (low-sodium)
- 1/4 cup spinach, chopped
- 1 teaspoon olive oil
- Italian seasoning for garnish

Cooking Instructions:

1. Preheat the oven to 375°F (190°C).
2. In a baking dish, layer zucchini slices, ricotta, mozzarella, tomato sauce, and spinach.
3. Repeat layers and finish with a sprinkle of Italian seasoning.
4. Bake for 30 minutes or until the top is golden and bubbly.

Nutritional Information:

- Calories: 280
- Protein: 18g
- Carbohydrates: 12g
- Fat: 18g
- Fiber: 3g

Tips for Recipe Modification:

- Use low-fat ricotta for a lighter version.
- Add sliced mushrooms or bell peppers for extra veggies.

CABBAGE AND TURKEY STIR-FRY

Prep/Cook Time: 30 minutes

Ingredients (for one serving):

- 1 cup green cabbage, shredded
- 4 ounces ground turkey
- 1/4 cup carrots, julienned
- 1/4 cup snow peas
- 1 tablespoon low-sodium soy sauce
- 1 tablespoon hoisin sauce
- 1 teaspoon sesame oil

Cooking Instructions:

1. In a wok or skillet, cook ground turkey until browned.
2. Add cabbage, carrots, and snow peas. Stir-fry until vegetables are tender-crisp.
3. Drizzle with soy sauce, hoisin sauce, and sesame oil. Toss to combine.

Nutritional Information:

- Calories: 290
- Protein: 25g
- Carbohydrates: 20g
- Fat: 12g
- Fiber: 5g

Tips for Recipe Modification:

- Use lean ground chicken or tofu.
- Serve over cauliflower rice for a low-carb option.

SALMON AND QUINOA BOWL

Prep/Cook Time: 25 minutes

Ingredients (for one serving):

- 4 ounces salmon fillet
- 1/2 cup cooked quinoa
- 1/4 cup cucumber, diced
- 1/4 cup cherry tomatoes, halved
- 1 tablespoon olive oil
- Fresh lemon juice
- Dill for garnish

Cooking Instructions:

1. Grill or bake salmon until fully cooked.
2. In a bowl, combine cooked quinoa, cucumber, and cherry tomatoes.
3. Top with grilled salmon, drizzle with olive oil, and squeeze fresh lemon juice. Garnish with dill.

Nutritional Information:

- Calories: 320
- Protein: 30g
- Carbohydrates: 20g
- Fat: 15g
- Fiber: 4g

Tips for Recipe Modification:

- Add a handful of baby spinach for extra greens.
- Substitute quinoa with brown rice or cauliflower rice.

Prep/Cook Time: 15 minutes

Ingredients (for one serving):

- 1 large tomato, sliced
- 1/2 cup fresh mozzarella, sliced
- Fresh basil leaves
- 1 tablespoon balsamic glaze
- Salt and pepper to taste

Cooking Instructions:

1. Arrange tomato and mozzarella slices on a plate.
2. Tuck fresh basil leaves between the slices.
3. Drizzle with balsamic glaze and season with salt and pepper.

Nutritional Information:

- Calories: 280
- Protein: 18g
- Carbohydrates: 10g
- Fat: 18g
- Fiber: 2g

Tips for Recipe Modification:

- Use cherry tomatoes for a bite-sized version.
- Add a drizzle of extra virgin olive oil for richness.

PESTO ZOODLES WITH CHERRY TOMATOES

Prep/Cook Time: 20 minutes

Ingredients (for one serving):

- 2 medium zucchinis, spiralized
- 2 tablespoons pesto sauce
- 1/2 cup cherry tomatoes, halved
- 1 tablespoon pine nuts, toasted
- Parmesan cheese for garnish

Cooking Instructions:

1. Spiralize zucchinis into noodle-like shapes.
2. In a pan, sauté zoodles with pesto until heated through.
3. Toss in cherry tomatoes and top with toasted pine nuts and Parmesan.

Nutritional Information:

- Calories: 250
- Protein: 8g
- Carbohydrates: 15g
- Fat: 18g
- Fiber: 4

Tips for Recipe Modification:

- Add grilled chicken for extra protein.
- Use a mix of green and yellow zucchini for color.

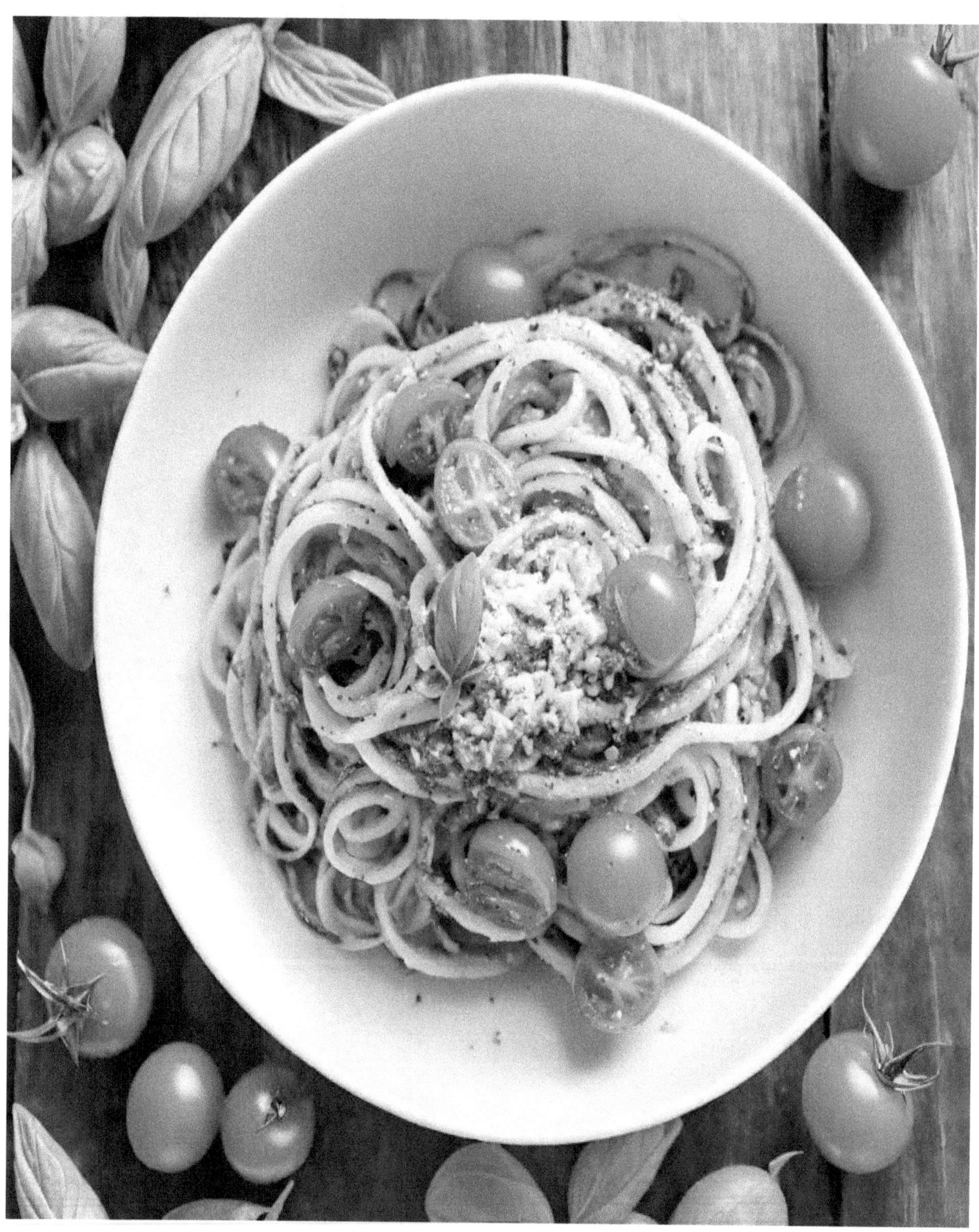

BAKED LEMON HERB TILAPIA

Prep/Cook Time: 25 minutes

Ingredients (for one serving):

- 6 ounces tilapia fillet
- 1 tablespoon olive oil
- 1 teaspoon lemon zest
- 1 teaspoon fresh herbs (parsley, dill)
- Salt and pepper to taste

Cooking Instructions:

1. Preheat the oven to 375°F (190°C).
2. Place tilapia on a baking sheet, drizzle with olive oil, and sprinkle with lemon zest, herbs, salt, and pepper.
3. Bake for 15-18 minutes or until the fish flakes easily.

Nutritional Information:

- Calories: 250
- Protein: 30g
- Carbohydrates: 0g
- Fat: 14g
- Fiber: 0g

Tips for Recipe Modification:

- Substitute tilapia with another white fish.
- Serve with a side of steamed vegetables.

CAULIFLOWER RICE AND TURKEY STUFFED PEPPERS

Prep/Cook Time: 40 minutes

Ingredients (for one serving):

- 2 bell peppers, halved
- 4 ounces ground turkey
- 1/2 cup cauliflower rice
- 1/4 cup black beans, canned and rinsed
- 1/4 cup tomato sauce (low-sodium)
- 1 teaspoon taco seasoning

Cooking Instructions:

1. Preheat the oven to 375°F (190°C).
2. In a skillet, cook ground turkey until browned. Add cauliflower rice, black beans, tomato sauce, and taco seasoning.
3. Stuff bell peppers with the turkey mixture and bake for 25-30 minutes.

Nutritional Information:

- Calories: 320
- Protein: 25g
- Carbohydrates: 30g
- Fat: 12g
- Fiber: 7g

Tips for Recipe Modification:

- Use lean ground chicken as an alternative.
- Top with a dollop of Greek yogurt instead of sour cream.

SALMON AND ASPARAGUS FOIL PACKETS

Prep/Cook Time: 30 minutes

Ingredients (for one serving):

- 6 ounces salmon fillet
- 1/2 bunch asparagus, trimmed
- 1 tablespoon olive oil
- Lemon slices
- Salt and pepper to taste

Cooking Instructions:

1. Preheat the oven to 400°F (200°C).
2. Place salmon and asparagus on a sheet of foil. Drizzle with olive oil, season with salt and pepper, and top with lemon slices.
3. Seal the foil into packets and bake for 20-25 minutes.

Nutritional Information:

- Calories: 300
- Protein: 25g
- Carbohydrates: 8g
- Fat: 18g
- Fiber: 4g

Tips for Recipe Modification:

- Substitute asparagus with green beans or zucchini.
- Sprinkle with chopped dill for added freshness.

Prep/Cook Time: 45 minutes

Ingredients (for one serving):

- 1 medium eggplant, sliced lengthwise
- 1/2 cup ricotta cheese
- 1/4 cup mozzarella cheese, shredded
- 1/4 cup tomato sauce (low-sodium)
- 1/4 cup spinach, chopped
- 1 teaspoon olive oil
- Italian seasoning for garnish

Cooking Instructions:

1. Preheat the oven to 375°F (190°C).
2. In a baking dish, layer eggplant slices, ricotta, mozzarella, tomato sauce, and spinach.
3. Repeat layers and finish with a sprinkle of Italian seasoning.
4. Bake for 30 minutes or until the top is golden and bubbly.

Nutritional Information:

- Calories: 280
- Protein: 18g
- Carbohydrates: 12g
- Fat: 18g
- Fiber: 3g

Tips for Recipe Modification:

- Use low-fat ricotta for a lighter version.
- Add sliced mushrooms or bell peppers for extra veggies.

Prep/Cook Time: 30 minutes

Ingredients (for one serving):

- 6 ounces chicken breast
- 1/2 cup cooked quinoa
- 1 cup mixed greens
- 1/4 cup cherry tomatoes, halved
- 1/4 cup cucumber, diced
- 1 tablespoon balsamic vinaigrette

Cooking Instructions:

1. Season chicken with salt and pepper and grill until fully cooked.
2. In a bowl, combine quinoa, mixed greens, cherry tomatoes, and cucumber.
3. Slice grilled chicken and place on top of the salad. Drizzle with balsamic vinaigrette.

Nutritional Information:

- Calories: 320
- Protein: 30g
- Carbohydrates: 20g
- Fat: 15g
- Fiber: 4g

Tips for Recipe Modification:

- Add feta or goat cheese for extra flavor.
- Use a lemon vinaigrette for a citrusy twist.

LEMON GARLIC SHRIMP AND BROCCOLI STIR-FRY

Prep/Cook Time: 20 minutes

Ingredients (for one serving):

- 4 ounces shrimp, peeled and deveined
- 1 cup broccoli florets
- 1/2 cup snap peas
- 1 tablespoon olive oil
- 1 teaspoon lemon zest
- 1 clove garlic, minced

Cooking Instructions:

1. In a wok or skillet, heat olive oil and sauté shrimp until pink.
2. Add broccoli and snap peas, stir-frying until vegetables are tender.
3. Stir in lemon zest and minced garlic.

Nutritional Information:

- Calories: 250
- Protein: 25g
- Carbohydrates: 10g
- Fat: 14g
- Fiber: 4g

Tips for Recipe Modification:

- Serve over cauliflower rice for a low-carb option.
- Include a dash of low-sodium soy sauce for flavor.

Prep/Cook Time: 40 minutes

Ingredients (for one serving):

- 2 bell peppers, halved
- 1/2 cup cooked quinoa
- 1/4 cup black beans, canned and rinsed
- 1/4 cup corn kernels
- 1/4 cup tomato sauce (low-sodium)
- 1 teaspoon cumin powder

Cooking Instructions:

1. Preheat the oven to 375°F (190°C).
2. In a bowl, mix cooked quinoa, black beans, corn, tomato sauce, and cumin.
3. Stuff bell peppers with the quinoa mixture and bake for 25-30 minutes.

Nutritional Information:

- Calories: 320
- Protein: 15g
- Carbohydrates: 60g
- Fat: 4g
- Fiber: 10g

Tips for Recipe Modification:

- Top with avocado slices for creaminess.
- Sprinkle with chopped cilantro for freshness.

TURKEY AND VEGETABLE SKEWERS WITH YOGURT SAUCE

Prep/Cook Time: 25 minutes

Ingredients (for one serving):

- 4 ounces ground turkey
- 1/2 bell pepper, diced
- 1/2 zucchini, sliced
- 1 tablespoon olive oil
- 1 teaspoon dried oregano
- Salt and pepper to taste
- Yogurt sauce for dipping

Cooking Instructions:

1. In a bowl, mix ground turkey, bell pepper, zucchini, olive oil, dried oregano, salt, and pepper.
2. Thread the mixture onto skewers and grill until turkey is fully cooked.
3. Serve with yogurt sauce for dipping.

Nutritional Information:

- Calories: 300
- Protein: 25g
- Carbohydrates: 10g
- Fat: 16g
- Fiber: 3g

Tips for Recipe Modification:

- Use lean ground chicken or beef.
- Make a tzatziki-style yogurt sauce with cucumber and dill.

Prep/Cook Time: 30 minutes

Ingredients (for one serving):

- 1 cup mixed vegetables (bell peppers, broccoli, snap peas)
- 1/2 cup firm tofu, cubed
- 1 tablespoon low-sodium soy sauce
- 1 tablespoon sesame oil
- 1 teaspoon ginger, grated
- 1 clove garlic, minced
- 1 cup cooked brown rice

Cooking Instructions:

1. In a wok or skillet, stir-fry tofu until golden brown.
2. Add mixed vegetables, ginger, and garlic. Stir-fry until vegetables are crisp-tender.
3. Drizzle with soy sauce and sesame oil. Toss to combine.
4. Serve over cooked brown rice.

Nutritional Information:

- Calories: 280
- Protein: 18g
- Carbohydrates: 45g
- Fat: 14g
- Fiber: 7g

Tips for Recipe Modification:

- Use quinoa instead of brown rice for variety.
- Add a sprinkle of sesame seeds for extra crunch.

MUSHROOM AND SPINACH RISOTTO

Prep/Cook Time: 40 minutes

Ingredients (for one serving):

- 1/2 cup Arborio rice
- 1/4 cup mushrooms, sliced
- 1/4 cup spinach, chopped
- 1/4 cup Parmesan cheese, grated
- 1/4 cup white wine (optional)
- 1 tablespoon olive oil
- 1 clove garlic, minced
- 4 cups low-sodium vegetable broth, warmed

Cooking Instructions:

1. In a pan, sauté mushrooms and garlic in olive oil until mushrooms are browned.
2. Add Arborio rice and stir until lightly toasted.
3. Pour in white wine and cook until mostly evaporated.
4. Gradually add warm vegetable broth, stirring constantly until rice is creamy and cooked.
5. Stir in chopped spinach and Parmesan cheese before serving.

Nutritional Information:

- Calories: 350
- Protein: 10g
- Carbohydrates: 50g
- Fat: 12g
- Fiber: 4g

Tips for Recipe Modification:

- Use whole-grain Arborio rice for added fiber.
- Add a touch of nutmeg for extra depth of flavor.

Prep/Cook Time: 30 minutes

Ingredients (for one serving):

- 6 ounces chicken breast
- 1/2 cup cooked quinoa
- 1 cup broccoli florets
- 1 tablespoon olive oil
- Lemon juice
- Salt and pepper to taste

Cooking Instructions:

1. Season chicken with salt and pepper and grill until fully cooked.
2. In a pan, sauté broccoli in olive oil until tender-crisp.
3. Assemble the bowl with cooked quinoa, grilled chicken, and sautéed broccoli. Drizzle with lemon juice.

Nutritional Information:

- Calories: 320
- Protein: 30g
- Carbohydrates: 20g
- Fat: 15g
- Fiber: 4g

Tips for Recipe Modification:

- Add a sprinkle of crushed red pepper for a kick.
- Substitute broccoli with asparagus or green beans.

VEGETARIAN LENTIL AND VEGETABLE CURRY

Prep/Cook Time: 45 minutes

Ingredients (for one serving):

- 1/2 cup dry lentils, rinsed
- 1/4 cup carrots, diced
- 1/4 cup bell peppers, diced
- 1/4 cup onion, finely chopped
- 1 clove garlic, minced
- 1/4 cup coconut milk
- 1 tablespoon curry powder
- 1 tablespoon olive oil

Cooking Instructions:

1. In a pot, sauté onions and garlic in olive oil until softened.
2. Add lentils, carrots, bell peppers, coconut milk, and curry powder. Simmer until lentils are tender.
3. Serve over cooked brown rice or quinoa.

Nutritional Information:

- Calories: 280
- Protein: 15g
- Carbohydrates: 40g
- Fat: 8g
- Fiber: 12g

Tips for Recipe Modification:

- Add a handful of spinach or kale for extra greens.
- Garnish with fresh cilantro before serving.

MEDITERRANEAN GRILLED VEGETABLE SKEWERS

Prep/Cook Time: 30 minutes

Ingredients (for one serving):

- 1/2 zucchini, sliced
- 1/2 bell pepper, diced
- 1/2 red onion, cut into wedges
- Cherry tomatoes
- 1 tablespoon olive oil
- 1 teaspoon dried oregano
- Salt and pepper to taste

Cooking Instructions:

1. Thread zucchini, bell pepper, red onion, and cherry tomatoes onto skewers.
2. Mix olive oil, dried oregano, salt, and pepper. Brush onto skewers.
3. Grill until vegetables are tender and slightly charred.

Nutritional Information:

- Calories: 250
- Protein: 5g
- Carbohydrates: 25g
- Fat: 15g
- Fiber: 6g

Tips for Recipe Modification:

- Serve with a side of Greek yogurt or tzatziki.
- Add a squeeze of lemon juice before serving.

Prep/Cook Time: 25 minutes

Ingredients (for one serving):

- 1 cup mixed vegetables (broccoli, snap peas, carrots)
- 1/2 cup brown rice, cooked
- 4 ounces shrimp, peeled and deveined
- 1 tablespoon low-sodium soy sauce
- 1 tablespoon sesame oil
- 1 teaspoon ginger, grated
- 1 clove garlic, minced
- Green onions for garnish

Cooking Instructions:

1. In a wok or skillet, heat sesame oil and sauté shrimp until pink. Remove and set aside.
2. Stir-fry mixed vegetables in the same pan until they are crisp-tender.
3. Add grated ginger and minced garlic to the vegetables, followed by the cooked shrimp.
4. Pour in low-sodium soy sauce and toss until everything is well-coated.
5. Serve the stir-fry over a bed of cooked brown rice and garnish with chopped green onions.

Nutritional Information:

- Calories: 300
- Protein: 20g
- Carbohydrates: 40g
- Fat: 8g
- Fiber: 6g

Tips for Recipe Modification:

- Substitute shrimp with tofu or chicken for variation.
- Increase the variety of vegetables, such as adding bell peppers or water chestnuts.

TOMATO BASIL GRILLED CHICKEN

Prep/Cook Time: 30 minutes

Ingredients (for one serving):

- 6 ounces chicken breast
- 1 large tomato, sliced
- Fresh basil leaves
- 1 tablespoon olive oil
- Balsamic glaze for drizzling
- Salt and pepper to taste

Cooking Instructions:

1. Preheat the grill or grill pan.
2. Season chicken with salt and pepper and grill until fully cooked.
3. In the last few minutes of grilling, add tomato slices to the grill until they are slightly charred.
4. Arrange grilled chicken on a plate, top with grilled tomatoes, fresh basil leaves, and drizzle with olive oil and balsamic glaze.

Nutritional Information:

- Calories: 320
- Protein: 35g
- Carbohydrates: 5g
- Fat: 18g
- Fiber: 2g

Tips for Recipe Modification:

- Use cherry tomatoes for a quicker cooking time.
- Sprinkle with crumbled feta for added flavor.

LEMON HERB BAKED CHICKEN THIGHS

Prep/Cook Time: 35 minutes

Ingredients (for one serving):

- 4 bone-in, skin-on chicken thighs
- 1 tablespoon olive oil
- 1 teaspoon lemon zest
- 1 teaspoon fresh herbs (thyme, rosemary)
- 1 clove garlic, minced
- Salt and pepper to taste

Cooking Instructions:

1. Preheat the oven to 400°F (200°C).
2. Pat the chicken thighs dry with a paper towel and place them on a baking sheet.
3. In a bowl, mix olive oil, lemon zest, fresh herbs, minced garlic, salt, and pepper.
4. Rub the herb mixture over the chicken thighs.
5. Bake for 25-30 minutes or until the chicken reaches an internal temperature of 165°F (74°C).

Nutritional Information:

- Calories: 350
- Protein: 30g
- Carbohydrates: 0g
- Fat: 24g
- Fiber: 0g

Tips for Recipe Modification:

- Use boneless, skinless chicken thighs for a lighter option.
- Serve with a side of steamed green beans or asparagus.

Prep/Cook Time: 25 minutes

Ingredients (for one serving):

- 4 ounces chicken breast, thinly sliced
- 1 cup green cabbage, shredded
- 1/4 cup carrots, julienned
- 1/4 cup red bell pepper, sliced
- 1 tablespoon low-sodium soy sauce
- 1 tablespoon sesame oil
- 1 teaspoon ginger, grated

Cooking Instructions:

1. In a wok or skillet, heat sesame oil and sauté chicken until browned.
2. Add shredded cabbage, julienned carrots, and sliced red bell pepper. Stir-fry until vegetables are tender.
3. Drizzle with low-sodium soy sauce and add grated ginger. Toss until well combined.

Nutritional Information:

- Calories: 280
- Protein: 25g
- Carbohydrates: 15g
- Fat: 14g
- Fiber: 6g

Tips for Recipe Modification:

- Add a handful of bean sprouts for extra crunch.
- Serve over cauliflower rice for a low-carb option.

STUFFED PORTOBELLO MUSHROOMS WITH TURKEY

Prep/Cook Time: 30 minutes

Ingredients (for one serving):

- 2 large portobello mushrooms, stems removed
- 4 ounces ground turkey
- 1/4 cup quinoa, cooked
- 1/4 cup spinach, chopped
- 1/4 cup feta cheese, crumbled
- 1 tablespoon olive oil
- Italian seasoning for garnish

Cooking Instructions:

1. Preheat the oven to 375°F (190°C).
2. In a skillet, cook ground turkey until browned. Add cooked quinoa, chopped spinach, and feta cheese.
3. Stuff portobello mushrooms with the turkey mixture and bake for 20-25 minutes.
4. Sprinkle with Italian seasoning before serving.

Nutritional Information:

- Calories: 320
- Protein: 25g
- Carbohydrates: 20g
- Fat: 18g
- Fiber: 4g

Tips for Recipe Modification:

- Use ground chicken or beef as an alternative.
- Top with a dollop of Greek yogurt for creaminess.

MEDITERRANEAN SHRIMP AND QUINOA BOWL

Prep/Cook Time: 30 minutes

Ingredients (for one serving):

- 4 ounces shrimp, peeled and deveined
- 1/2 cup cooked quinoa
- 1/4 cup cherry tomatoes, halved
- 1/4 cup cucumber, diced
- Kalamata olives, pitted
- Feta cheese, crumbled
- Olive oil and lemon juice dressing

Cooking Instructions:

1. In a pan, sauté shrimp until pink and cooked through.
2. In a bowl, combine cooked quinoa, cherry tomatoes, cucumber, Kalamata olives, and feta cheese.
3. Top the quinoa mixture with the cooked shrimp.
4. Drizzle with olive oil and lemon juice dressing before serving.

Nutritional Information:

- Calories: 300
- Protein: 20g
- Carbohydrates: 30g
- Fat: 14g
- Fiber: 5g

- Add chopped fresh parsley for brightness.
- Substitute feta with goat cheese for a different flavor.

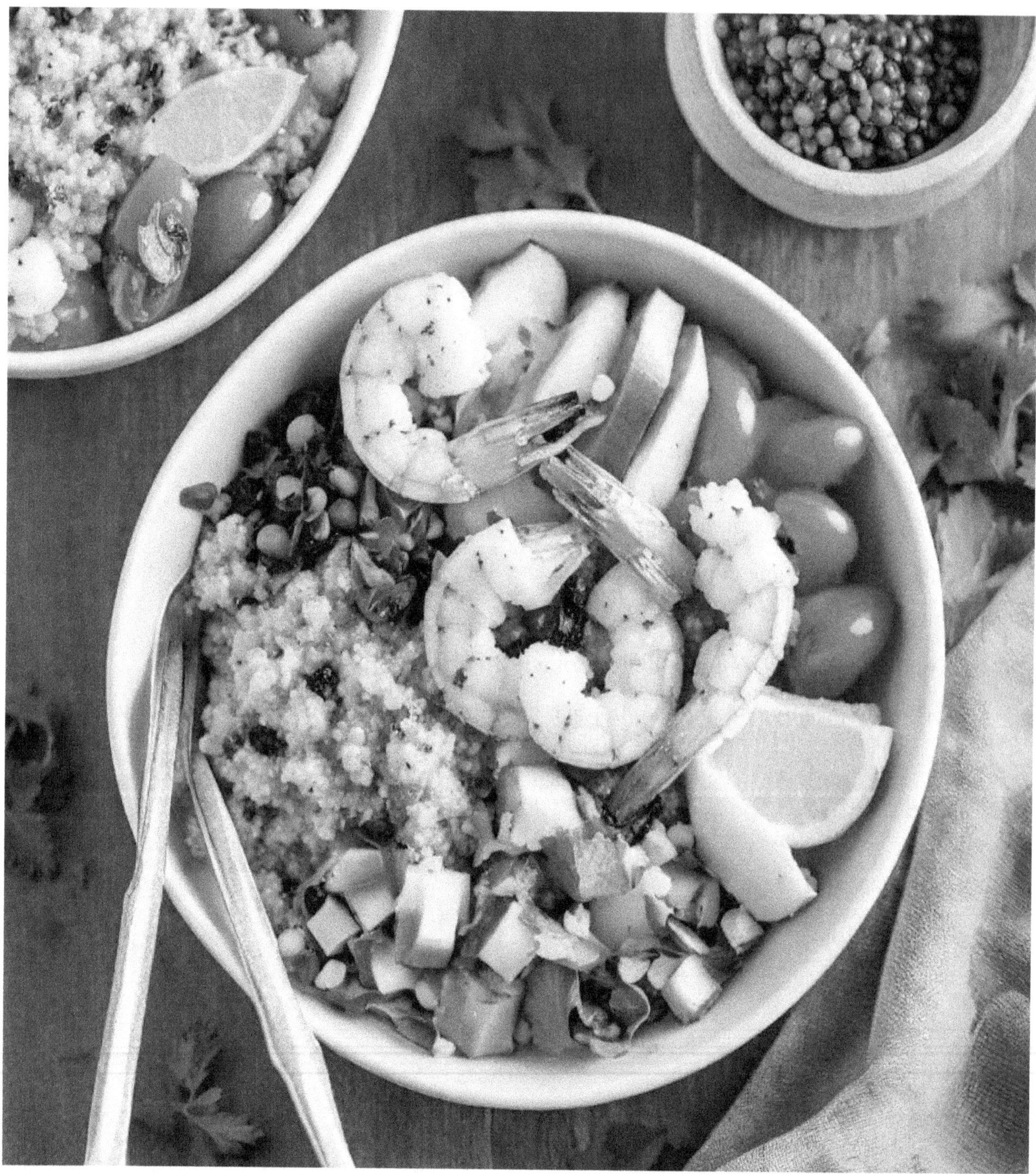

HUMMUS AND VEGGIE STICKS

Prep Time: 10 minutes

Ingredients (for one serving):

- 1/2 cup hummus
- Carrot sticks, cucumber slices, and bell pepper strips for dipping

Instructions:

1. Arrange hummus in a small bowl.
2. Wash and cut carrot sticks, cucumber slices, and bell pepper strips.
3. Dip the veggies into hummus and enjoy!

Nutritional Information:

- Calories: 150
- Protein: 6g
- Carbohydrates: 18g
- Fat: 7g
- Fiber: 5g

Tips for Recipe Modification:

- Choose a low-sodium hummus for a kidney-friendly option.
- Add a sprinkle of paprika or cumin for extra flavor.

Prep Time: 15 minutes

Ingredients (for one serving):

- 1 small cucumber, sliced
- 1/2 can tuna, drained
- 1 tablespoon Greek yogurt
- Cherry tomatoes for garnish

Instructions:

1. In a bowl, mix drained tuna with Greek yogurt.
2. Place a spoonful of tuna mixture on each cucumber slice.
3. Garnish with halved cherry tomatoes.

Nutritional Information:

- Calories: 180
- Protein: 20g
- Carbohydrates: 5g
- Fat: 9g
- Fiber: 2g

Tips for Recipe Modification:

- Choose tuna canned in water for a lower sodium option.
- Add a squeeze of lemon juice for freshness.

AVOCADO AND TOMATO SALSA

Prep Time: 10 minutes

Ingredients (for one serving):

- 1/2 avocado, diced
- 1/2 cup cherry tomatoes, diced
- 1 tablespoon red onion, finely chopped
- Fresh cilantro, chopped
- Lime juice for drizzling

Cooking Instructions:

1. In a bowl, combine diced avocado, cherry tomatoes, red onion, and cilantro.
2. Drizzle with lime juice and toss gently.
3. Serve with whole-grain crackers or sliced cucumber.

Nutritional Information:

- Calories: 160
- Protein: 2g
- Carbohydrates: 12g
- Fat: 13g
- Fiber: 5g

Tips for Recipe Modification:

- Adjust the amount of lime juice to taste.
- Sprinkle with a pinch of salt if desired.

EGG SALAD LETTUCE WRAPS

Prep Time: 15 minutes

Ingredients (for one serving):

- 2 hard-boiled eggs, chopped
- 1 tablespoon mayonnaise (low-fat)
- 1 teaspoon Dijon mustard
- Lettuce leaves for wrapping

Cooking Instructions:

1. In a bowl, mix chopped hard-boiled eggs with mayonnaise and Dijon mustard.
2. Spoon the egg salad onto lettuce leaves.
3. Roll the lettuce leaves to form wraps.

Nutritional Information:

- Calories: 180
- Protein: 14g
- Carbohydrates: 2g
- Fat: 13g
- Fiber: 1g

Tips for Recipe Modification:

- Use Greek yogurt instead of mayonnaise for a lighter option.
- Add chopped celery for extra crunch.

BAKED PARMESAN ZUCCHINI CHIPS

Prep Time: 20 minutes

Ingredients (for one serving):

- 1 medium zucchini, thinly sliced
- 1 tablespoon olive oil
- 2 tablespoons grated Parmesan cheese
- Garlic powder and black pepper to taste

Cooking Instructions:

1. Preheat the oven to 400°F (200°C).
2. Toss zucchini slices with olive oil, Parmesan cheese, garlic powder, and black pepper.
3. Arrange the slices on a baking sheet and bake for 15-20 minutes until crispy.

Nutritional Information:

- Calories: 120
- Protein: 5g
- Carbohydrates: 6g
- Fat: 9g
- Fiber: 2g

Tips for Recipe Modification:

1. Use a mix of Parmesan and nutritional yeast for a cheesy flavor.
2. Serve with a side of tzatziki for dipping.

Prep Time: 10 minutes

Ingredients (for one serving):

- 1 banana, sliced
- 2 tablespoons peanut butter (unsweetened)
- Chopped nuts or shredded coconut for topping

Cooking Instructions:

1. Spread peanut butter on banana slices.
2. Sprinkle with chopped nuts or shredded coconut.
3. Enjoy as is or refrigerate for a firmer texture.

Nutritional Information:

- Calories: 220
- Protein: 5g
- Carbohydrates: 25g
- Fat: 12g
- Fiber: 4g

Tips for Recipe Modification:

- Use almond or cashew butter as an alternative.
- Add a drizzle of honey for sweetness.

Prep Time: 5 minutes

Ingredients (for one serving):

- 1/2 cup low-fat cottage cheese
- 1/2 cup fresh pineapple chunks
- Chopped mint for garnish

Cooking Instructions:

1. In a bowl, combine cottage cheese and fresh pineapple chunks.
2. Garnish with chopped mint.

Nutritional Information:

- Calories: 160
- Protein: 14g
- Carbohydrates: 22g
- Fat: 2g
- Fiber: 2g

Tips for Recipe Modification:

- Use canned pineapple in juice (not syrup) for convenience.
- Sprinkle with a pinch of cinnamon for added flavor.

Prep Time: 15 minutes

Ingredients (for one serving):

- 1/2 cup dried cherries, chopped
- 1/4 cup almonds, finely chopped
- 1 tablespoon chia seeds
- 1 tablespoon almond butter (unsweetened)
- 1 tablespoon honey

Instructions:

1. In a bowl, combine dried cherries, almonds, chia seeds, almond butter, and honey.
2. Mix until well combined.
3. Form the mixture into bite-sized balls.

Nutritional Information:

- Calories: 180
- Protein: 4g
- Carbohydrates: 25g
- Fat: 9g
- Fiber: 4g

Tips for Recipe Modification:

- Add a scoop of protein powder for an extra protein boost.
- Roll the bites in shredded coconut for a different texture.

SMOKED SALMON CUCUMBER ROLLS

Prep Time: 15 minutes

Ingredients (for one serving):

- 4 slices smoked salmon
- 1/2 cucumber, thinly sliced
- Cream cheese (low-fat) for spreading

Cooking Instructions:

1. Lay out smoked salmon slices.
2. Spread a thin layer of cream cheese on each slice.
3. Place cucumber slices on top and roll up.

Nutritional Information:

- Calories: 180
- Protein: 15g
- Carbohydrates: 3g
- Fat: 12g
- Fiber: 1g

Tips for Recipe Modification:

- Add a squeeze of lemon juice for freshness.
- Sprinkle with chopped dill for extra flavor.

STUFFED CHERRY TOMATOES WITH TUNA

Prep Time: 10 minutes

Ingredients (for one serving):

- Cherry tomatoes, halved
- 1/2 can tuna, drained
- 1 tablespoon Greek yogurt
- Chopped chives for garnish

Cooking Instructions:

1. In a bowl, mix drained tuna with Greek yogurt.
2. Spoon the tuna mixture into halved cherry tomatoes.
3. Garnish with chopped chives.

Nutritional Information:

- Calories: 160
- Protein: 18g
- Carbohydrates: 4g
- Fat: 8g
- Fiber: 1g

Tips for Recipe Modification:

- Add a pinch of black pepper or paprika for spice.
- Use flavored tuna for variety.

BAKED APPLE CHIPS

Prep Time: 15 minutes

Ingredients (for one serving):

- 1 apple, thinly sliced
- Cinnamon for sprinkling

Cooking Instructions:

1. Preheat the oven to 200°F (93°C).
2. Arrange apple slices on a baking sheet.
3. Sprinkle with cinnamon and bake for 2-3 hours until crispy.

Nutritional Information:

- Calories: 90
- Protein: 0g
- Carbohydrates: 25g
- Fat: 0g
- Fiber: 4g

Tips for Recipe Modification:

- Try different apple varieties for diverse flavors.
- Serve with a side of unsweetened yogurt for dipping.

Prep Time: 10 minutes

Ingredients (for one serving):

- 1 cup edamame, boiled and drained
- 1 teaspoon olive oil
- Chili powder and sea salt to taste

Cooking Instructions:

1. In a bowl, toss boiled edamame with olive oil, chili powder, and sea salt.
2. Serve warm or at room temperature.

Nutritional Information:

- Calories: 140
- Protein: 12g
- Carbohydrates: 9g
- Fat: 7g
- Fiber: 5g

Tips for Recipe Modification:

- Use a blend of spices for a more complex flavor.
- Squeeze a lime wedge over the edamame for acidity.

QUINOA AND CRANBERRY STUFFED DATES

Prep Time: 15 minutes

Ingredients (for one serving):

- 4 Medjool dates, pitted
- 1/4 cup cooked quinoa
- 1 tablespoon dried cranberries
- Almond butter for drizzling

Cooking Instructions:

1. In a bowl, mix cooked quinoa and dried cranberries.
2. Stuff each date with the quinoa mixture.
3. Drizzle with almond butter before serving.

Nutritional Information:

- Calories: 200
- Protein: 4g
- Carbohydrates: 45g
- Fat: 3g
- Fiber: 5g

Tips for Recipe Modification:

- Add a pinch of cinnamon or nutmeg for warmth.
- Substitute almond butter with cashew or peanut butter.

Prep Time: 15 minutes

Ingredients (for one serving):

- Cherry tomatoes
- Fresh mozzarella balls
- Fresh basil leaves
- Balsamic glaze for drizzling

Cooking Instructions:

1. Thread cherry tomatoes, fresh mozzarella balls, and basil leaves onto small skewers.
2. Arrange the skewers on a serving plate.
3. Drizzle with balsamic glaze before serving.

Nutritional Information:

- Calories: 180
- Protein: 8g
- Carbohydrates: 5g
- Fat: 14g
- Fiber: 2g

Tips for Recipe Modification:

- Use reduced-fat mozzarella for a lighter option.
- Add a sprinkle of salt and black pepper to taste.

WALNUT AND BERRY SALAD

Prep Time: 10 minutes

Ingredients (for one serving):

- Mixed berries (strawberries, blueberries, raspberries)
- 1/4 cup walnuts, chopped
- Mixed salad greens
- Balsamic vinaigrette for dressing

Cooking Instructions:

1. In a bowl, combine mixed berries, chopped walnuts, and salad greens.
2. Drizzle with balsamic vinaigrette and toss gently.
3. Serve immediately.

Nutritional Information:

- Calories: 220
- Protein: 5g
- Carbohydrates: 20g
- Fat: 15g
- Fiber: 4g

Tips for Recipe Modification:

- Add crumbled feta cheese for a savory twist.
- Substitute balsamic vinaigrette with olive oil and lemon juice.

Prep Time: 20 minutes

Ingredients (for one serving):

- 1/2 cup almonds
- 1 tablespoon honey
- 1 teaspoon ground cinnamon

Cooking Instructions:

1. Preheat the oven to 325°F (163°C).
2. In a bowl, toss almonds with honey and ground cinnamon.
3. Spread the almonds on a baking sheet and roast for 15-20 minutes, stirring occasionally.

Nutritional Information:

- Calories: 220
- Protein: 7g
- Carbohydrates: 14g
- Fat: 16g
- Fiber: 3g

Tips for Recipe Modification:

- Use a sugar substitute for a lower-sugar option.
- Sprinkle with a pinch of sea salt for a sweet and salty flavor.

MANGO SALSA WITH BAKED PITA CHIPS

Prep Time: 15 minutes

Ingredients (for one serving):

- 1 mango, diced
- 1/4 cup red onion, finely chopped
- 1/4 cup cilantro, chopped
- 1 jalapeño, finely diced (optional)
- Baked whole wheat pita chips for dipping

Cooking Instructions:

1. In a bowl, combine diced mango, chopped red onion, cilantro, and jalapeño.
2. Mix well to create the salsa.
3. Serve with baked whole wheat pita chips.

Nutritional Information:

- Calories: 160
- Protein: 2g
- Carbohydrates: 38g
- Fat: 1g
- Fiber: 5g

Tips for Recipe Modification:

- Adjust the amount of jalapeño based on spice preference.
- Experiment with different fruit combinations, such as pineapple or peach.

KALE CHIPS

Prep Time: 15 minutes

Ingredients (for one serving):

- Fresh kale leaves, stems removed
- 1 tablespoon olive oil
- Sea salt and nutritional yeast for seasoning

Cooking Instructions:

1. Preheat the oven to 350°F (177°C).
2. Massage kale leaves with olive oil until coated.
3. Sprinkle with sea salt and nutritional yeast.
4. Arrange on a baking sheet and bake for 10-15 minutes until crispy.

Nutritional Information:

- Calories: 100
- Protein: 5g
- Carbohydrates: 8g
- Fat: 7g
- Fiber: 3g

Tips for Recipe Modification:

- Experiment with different seasonings, such as garlic powder or paprika.
- Store in an airtight container for freshness.

WATERMELON AND FETA SKEWERS

Prep Time: 10 minutes

Ingredients (for one serving):

- Watermelon cubes
- Feta cheese, cubed
- Fresh mint leaves
- Balsamic glaze for drizzling

Cooking Instructions:

1. Thread watermelon cubes, feta cheese, and fresh mint leaves onto small skewers.
2. Arrange the skewers on a serving plate.
3. Drizzle with balsamic glaze before serving.

Nutritional Information:

- Calories: 150
- Protein: 4g
- Carbohydrates: 20g
- Fat: 7g
- Fiber: 2g

Tips for Recipe Modification:

- Use reduced-fat feta for a lighter option.
- Add a sprinkle of black pepper for extra flavor.

Prep Time: 5 minutes (plus chilling time)

Ingredients (for one serving):

- 2 tablespoons chia seeds
- 1/2 cup almond milk (unsweetened)
- Mixed berries for topping
- Drizzle of honey (optional)

Cooking Instructions:

1. In a jar, mix chia seeds and almond milk.
2. Stir well, cover, and refrigerate for at least 2 hours or overnight.
3. Top with mixed berries and drizzle with honey before serving.

Nutritional Information:

- Calories: 180
- Protein: 5g
- Carbohydrates: 20g
- Fat: 10g
- Fiber: 9g

Tips for Recipe Modification:

- Use coconut milk or Greek yogurt for a different base.
- Add a dash of vanilla extract for flavor.

CUCUMBER AND GREEK YOGURT DIP

Prep Time: 10 minutes

Ingredients (for one serving):

- 1/2 cucumber, finely diced
- 1/2 cup Greek yogurt
- Fresh dill, chopped
- Garlic powder to taste
- Whole-grain crackers for dipping

Cooking Instructions:

1. In a bowl, combine diced cucumber, Greek yogurt, chopped fresh dill, and garlic powder.
2. Mix well to create the dip.
3. Serve with whole-grain crackers.

Nutritional Information:

- Calories: 120
- Protein: 8g
- Carbohydrates: 15g
- Fat: 3g
- Fiber: 3g

Tips for Recipe Modification:

- Add a squeeze of lemon juice for brightness.
- Incorporate finely chopped red onion for added flavor.

Prep Time: 10 minutes

Ingredients (for one serving):

- 1/4 cup pumpkin seeds
- 1/4 cup dried cranberries
- 1/4 cup almonds
- Dark chocolate chips (optional)

Cooking Instructions:

1. In a bowl, combine pumpkin seeds, dried cranberries, and almonds.
2. Mix well to create the trail mix.
3. If desired, add dark chocolate chips for sweetness.

Nutritional Information:

- Calories: 180
- Protein: 6g
- Carbohydrates: 15g
- Fat: 12g
- Fiber: 4g

Tips for Recipe Modification:

- Use unsweetened dried fruit for lower sugar content.
- Experiment with different nuts, such as walnuts or pistachios.

SUN-DRIED TOMATO AND BASIL RICE CAKES

Prep Time: 10 minutes

Ingredients (for one serving):

- Brown rice cakes
- Sun-dried tomatoes, chopped
- Fresh basil leaves
- Olive tapenade for spreading

Cooking Instructions:

1. Spread olive tapenade on brown rice cakes.
2. Top with chopped sun-dried tomatoes and fresh basil leaves.
3. Serve as a flavorful and crunchy snack.

Nutritional Information:

- Calories: 150
- Protein: 3g
- Carbohydrates: 25g
- Fat: 4g
- Fiber: 2g

Tips for Recipe Modification:

- Use whole-grain rice cakes for added fiber.
- Drizzle with balsamic glaze for extra tanginess.

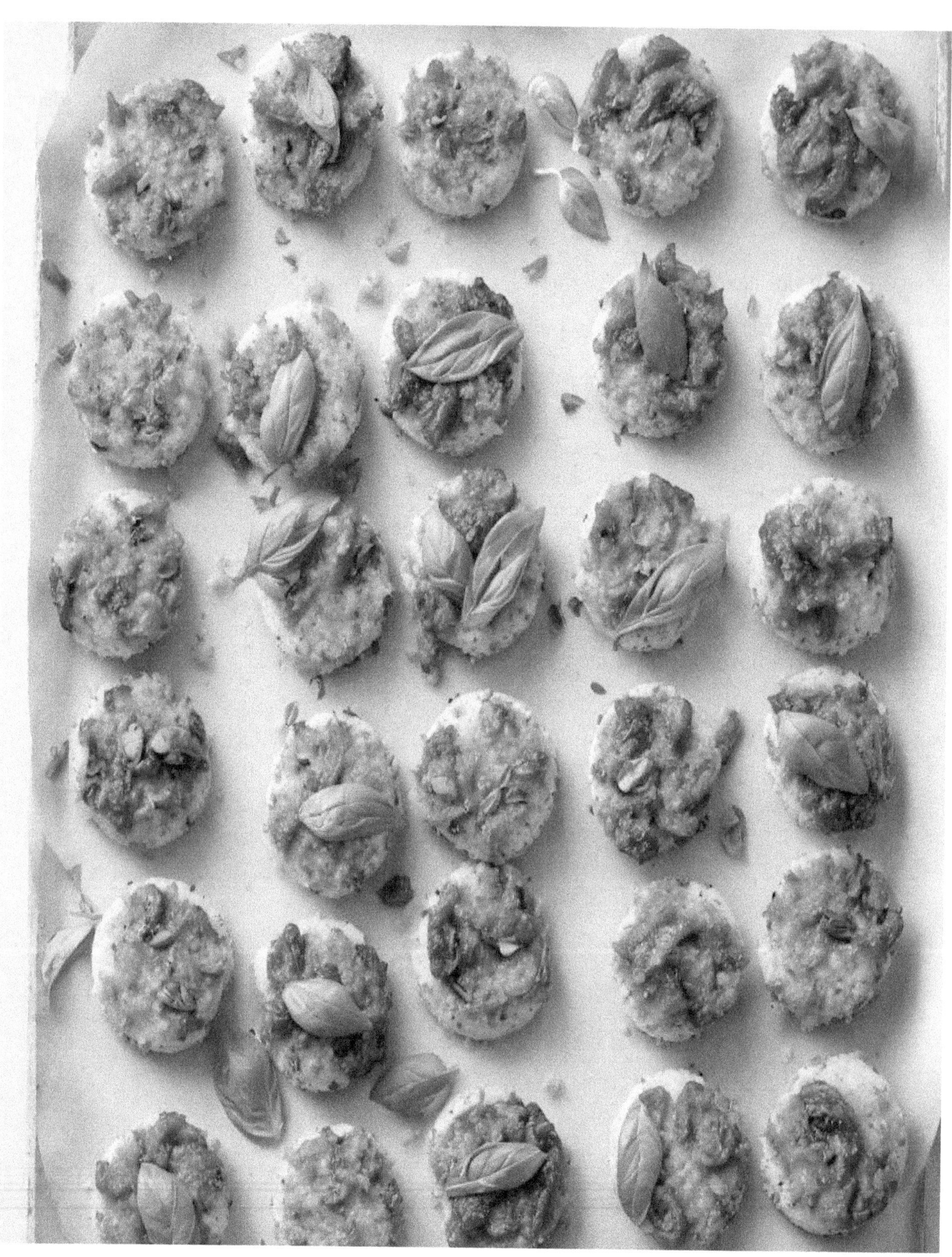

SOUPS

CHICKEN AND VEGETABLE QUINOA SOUP

Prep/Cook Time: 30 minutes

Ingredients (for one serving):

- 4 ounces chicken breast, cooked and shredded
- 1/4 cup quinoa, cooked
- 1 cup mixed vegetables (carrots, celery, green beans)
- 4 cups low-sodium chicken broth
- 1 teaspoon olive oil
- Salt and pepper to taste

Cooking Instructions:

1. In a pot, heat olive oil and sauté mixed vegetables until slightly softened.
2. Add shredded chicken, cooked quinoa, and chicken broth.
3. Season with salt and pepper and simmer for 15-20 minutes.
4. Serve hot.

Nutritional Information:

- Calories: 250
- Protein: 25g
- Carbohydrates: 20g
- Fat: 8g
- Fiber: 4g

- Add fresh herbs like thyme or rosemary for added flavor.
- Substitute chicken with turkey or tofu.

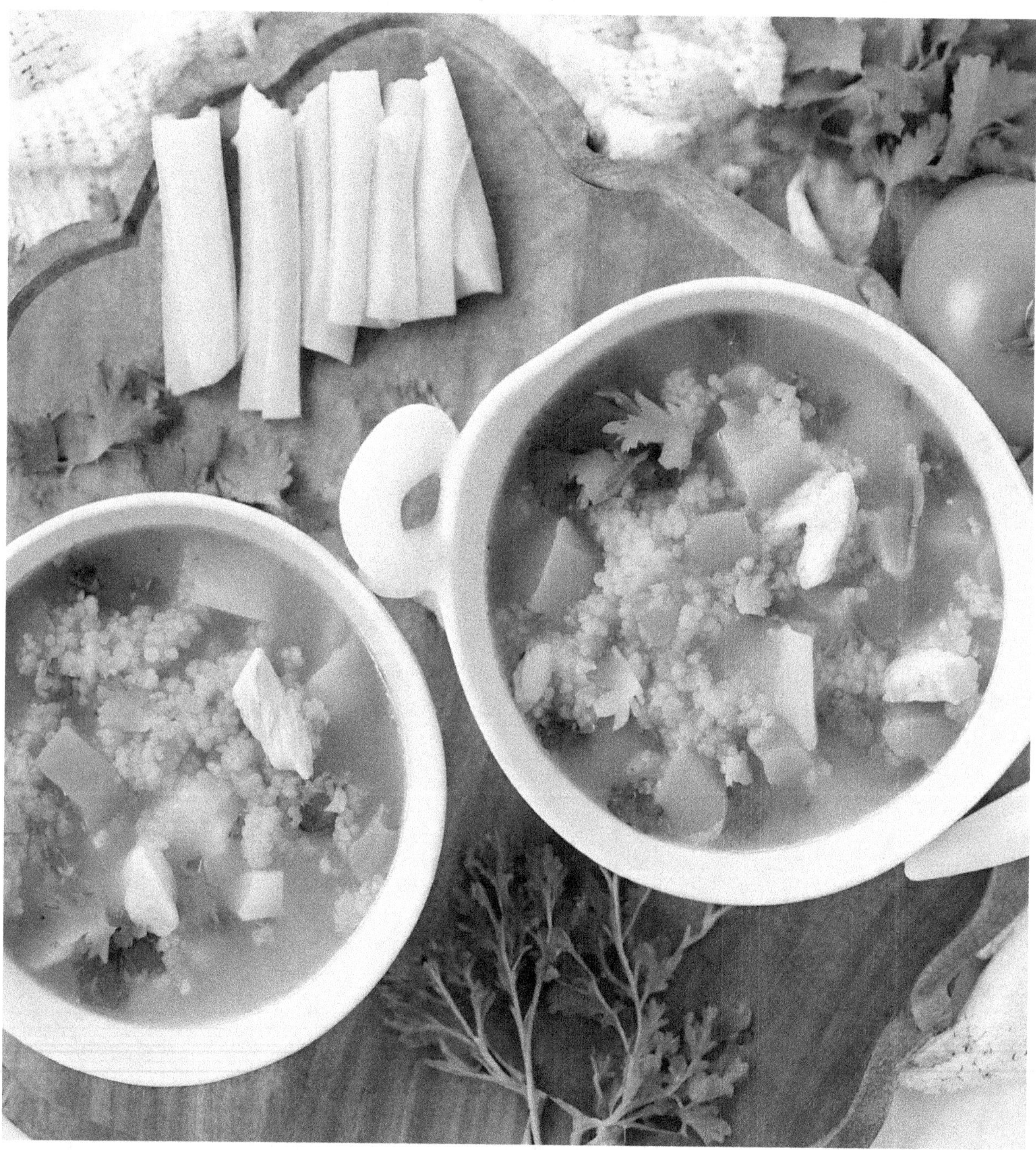

Prep/Cook Time: 40 minutes

Ingredients (for one serving):

- 1/2 cup dried lentils, rinsed
- 1 can (14 oz.) diced tomatoes
- 1/4 cup onion, chopped
- 2 cloves garlic, minced
- 1 teaspoon olive oil
- 4 cups vegetable broth
- Fresh basil leaves for garnish

Cooking Instructions:

1. In a pot, sauté onion and garlic in olive oil until fragrant.
2. Add lentils, diced tomatoes, and vegetable broth.
3. Bring to a boil, then simmer for 25-30 minutes until lentils are tender.
4. Garnish with fresh basil before serving.

Nutritional Information:

- Calories: 280
- Protein: 15g
- Carbohydrates: 45g
- Fat: 4g
- Fiber: 15g

Tips for Recipe Modification:

- Add a pinch of red pepper flakes for a hint of heat.
- Include diced carrots and celery for extra veggies.

MUSHROOM AND BARLEY SOUP

Prep/Cook Time: 45 minutes

Ingredients (for one serving):

- 1/2 cup pearl barley, rinsed
- 1 cup mushrooms, sliced
- 1/4 cup onion, finely chopped
- 2 cloves garlic, minced
- 4 cups vegetable broth
- 1 tablespoon olive oil
- Fresh parsley for garnish

Cooking Instructions:

1. In a pot, sauté onion and garlic in olive oil until softened.
2. Add sliced mushrooms and cook until they release their moisture.
3. Stir in pearl barley and vegetable broth. Simmer for 30-35 minutes.
4. Garnish with fresh parsley before serving.

Nutritional Information:

- Calories: 260
- Protein: 8g
- Carbohydrates: 50g
- Fat: 5g
- Fiber: 10g

Tips for Recipe Modification:

- Use a mix of wild mushrooms for a deeper flavor.
- Add a splash of balsamic vinegar for complexity.

Prep/Cook Time: 35 minutes

Ingredients (for one serving):

- 1/2 head cauliflower, chopped
- 1 leek, white and light green parts, sliced
- 1 clove garlic, minced
- 2 cups low-sodium vegetable broth
- 1/2 cup unsweetened almond milk
- 1 tablespoon olive oil
- Nutmeg and black pepper to taste

Cooking Instructions:

1. In a pot, sauté leek and garlic in olive oil until softened.
2. Add chopped cauliflower, vegetable broth, and almond milk. Simmer until cauliflower is tender.
3. Use an immersion blender to blend until smooth.
4. Season with nutmeg and black pepper. Serve warm.

Nutritional Information:

- Calories: 180
- Protein: 6g
- Carbohydrates: 20g
- Fat: 10g
- Fiber: 7g

Tips for Recipe Modification:

- Top with a dollop of Greek yogurt for creaminess.
- Garnish with chives or green onions.

SPINACH AND WHITE BEAN SOUP

Prep/Cook Time: 30 minutes

Ingredients (for one serving):

- 1 cup cannellini beans, cooked and drained
- 2 cups fresh spinach leaves
- 1/4 cup onion, diced
- 1 clove garlic, minced
- 4 cups low-sodium vegetable broth
- 1 tablespoon olive oil
- Lemon juice for a splash of freshness

Cooking Instructions:

1. In a pot, sauté onion and garlic in olive oil until translucent.
2. Add cooked cannellini beans, fresh spinach, and vegetable broth.
3. Simmer for 15-20 minutes until spinach wilts.
4. Finish with a splash of lemon juice before serving.

Nutritional Information:

- Calories: 220
- Protein: 10g
- Carbohydrates: 30g
- Fat: 7g
- Fiber: 10g

Tips for Recipe Modification:

- Stir in cooked quinoa for added protein and texture.
- Add a pinch of red pepper flakes for a subtle kick.

VEGETARIAN MINESTRONE SOUP

Prep/Cook Time: 40 minutes

Ingredients (for one serving):

- 1/2 cup whole wheat pasta, uncooked
- 1/2 cup kidney beans, cooked
- 1/4 cup zucchini, diced
- 1/4 cup carrots, sliced
- 2 cups low-sodium vegetable broth
- 1/4 cup onion, chopped
- 1 clove garlic, minced
- 1 tablespoon olive oil
- Italian seasoning and black pepper to taste

Cooking Instructions:

1. In a pot, sauté onion and garlic in olive oil until translucent.
2. Add diced zucchini, sliced carrots, kidney beans, and vegetable broth.
3. Bring to a boil, then add whole wheat pasta. Simmer until pasta is cooked.
4. Season with Italian seasoning and black pepper. Serve hot.

Nutritional Information:

- Calories: 260
- Protein: 10g
- Carbohydrates: 45g
- Fat: 5g
- Fiber: 8g

Tips for Recipe Modification:

- Use whole wheat orzo as a pasta alternative.
- Add spinach or kale for additional greens.

Prep/Cook Time: 30 minutes

Ingredients (for one serving):

- 4 ounces cooked chicken breast, shredded
- 1/4 cup brown rice, cooked
- 1/4 cup carrots, diced
- 1/4 cup celery, diced
- 4 cups low-sodium chicken broth
- 1 tablespoon olive oil
- Lemon juice and fresh dill for flavor

Cooking Instructions:

1. In a pot, sauté carrots and celery in olive oil until softened.
2. Add shredded chicken, cooked brown rice, and chicken broth.
3. Simmer for 15-20 minutes. Add lemon juice and fresh dill before serving.
4. Serve warm.

Nutritional Information:

- Calories: 280
- Protein: 25g
- Carbohydrates: 30g
- Fat: 8g
- Fiber: 4g

Tips for Recipe Modification:

- Substitute brown rice with quinoa for a different grain.
- Garnish with a slice of lemon for extra freshness.

Prep/Cook Time: 45 minutes

Ingredients (for one serving):

- 1/2 cup red lentils, rinsed
- 1 sweet potato, peeled and diced
- 1/4 cup onion, chopped
- 1 clove garlic, minced
- 4 cups vegetable broth
- 1 tablespoon olive oil
- Ground cumin and coriander to taste

Cooking Instructions:

- In a pot, sauté onion and garlic in olive oil until fragrant.
- Add diced sweet potato, red lentils, and vegetable broth.
- Simmer for 30-35 minutes until lentils and sweet potato are cooked.
- Season with ground cumin and coriander. Serve hot.

Nutritional Information:

- Calories: 250
- Protein: 12g
- Carbohydrates: 45g
- Fat: 5g
- Fiber: 10g

Tips for Recipe Modification:

- Garnish with chopped cilantro for added freshness.
- Add a pinch of smoked paprika for a smoky flavor.

Prep/Cook Time: 35 minutes

Ingredients (for one serving):

- 1 cup broccoli florets
- 1/4 cup onion, finely chopped
- 1 clove garlic, minced
- 2 cups low-sodium vegetable broth
- 1/2 cup shredded cheddar cheese
- 1/4 cup milk (unsweetened)
- 1 tablespoon olive oil
- Black pepper and nutmeg to taste

Cooking Instructions:

1. In a pot, sauté onion and garlic in olive oil until softened.
2. Add broccoli florets and vegetable broth. Simmer until broccoli is tender.
3. Use an immersion blender to blend until smooth.
4. Stir in shredded cheddar cheese, milk, black pepper, and nutmeg.
5. Serve hot.

Nutritional Information:

- Calories: 300
- Protein: 15g
- Carbohydrates: 25g
- Fat: 16g
- Fiber: 5g

Tips for Recipe Modification:

- Use sharp cheddar for a more intense flavor.
- Add a sprinkle of paprika for a touch of smokiness.

ROASTED VEGETABLE QUINOA SALAD

Prep Time: 25 minutes

Ingredients (for one serving):

- 1/2 cup cooked quinoa
- 1/2 cup cherry tomatoes, halved
- 1/4 cup bell peppers, diced
- 1/4 cup zucchini, sliced
- 1/4 cup red onion, thinly sliced
- Feta cheese for garnish
- Balsamic vinaigrette for dressing

Instructions:

1. In a bowl, combine cooked quinoa, cherry tomatoes, diced bell peppers, sliced zucchini, and thinly sliced red onion.
2. Drizzle with balsamic vinaigrette. Toss gently.
3. Garnish with crumbled feta cheese before serving.

Nutritional Information:

- Calories: 280
- Protein: 8g
- Carbohydrates: 40g
- Fat: 10g
- Fiber: 6g

Tips for Recipe Modification:

- Add grilled chicken for an extra protein boost.
- Use a mix of colorful bell peppers for visual appeal.

Prep Time: 15 minutes

Ingredients (for one serving):

- 1/2 avocado, diced
- 1/2 cup black beans, canned and rinsed
- 1/4 cup corn kernels (fresh or frozen)
- 1/4 cup red onion, finely chopped
- Cilantro, chopped
- Lime juice for dressing

Cooking Instructions:

1. In a bowl, combine diced avocado, black beans, corn kernels, chopped red onion, and cilantro.
2. Drizzle with lime juice. Toss gently.
3. Serve chilled.

Nutritional Information:

- Calories: 250
- Protein: 10g
- Carbohydrates: 30g
- Fat: 12g
- Fiber: 10g

Tips for Recipe Modification:

- Add diced tomatoes for extra juiciness.
- Include a pinch of cumin for a southwest flavor.

CRANBERRY AND ALMOND CHICKEN SALAD

Prep Time: 15 minutes

Ingredients (for one serving):

- 4 ounces grilled chicken breast, sliced
- Mixed salad greens
- 1/4 cup dried cranberries
- 1/4 cup almonds, sliced
- Raspberry vinaigrette for dressing

Instructions:

1. Arrange mixed salad greens on a plate.
2. Top with sliced grilled chicken, dried cranberries, and sliced almonds.
3. Drizzle with raspberry vinaigrette. Serve chilled.

Nutritional Information:

- Calories: 300
- Protein: 25g
- Carbohydrates: 20g
- Fat: 15g
- Fiber: 4g

Tips for Recipe Modification:

- Substitute dried cranberries with fresh berries for lower sugar.
- Add crumbled goat cheese for a creamy texture.

ASIAN-INSPIRED SHRIMP AND NOODLE SALAD

Prep Time: 20 minutes

Ingredients (for one serving):

- 4 ounces cooked shrimp
- 1/2 cup rice noodles, cooked
- 1/4 cup edamame, shelled
- 1/4 cup carrots, julienned
- 1/4 cup red cabbage, thinly sliced
- Sesame ginger dressing for flavor

Instructions:

1. In a bowl, combine cooked shrimp, rice noodles, shelled edamame, julienned carrots, and sliced red cabbage.
2. Drizzle with sesame ginger dressing. Toss gently.
3. Serve chilled.

Nutritional Information:

- Calories: 280
- Protein: 20g
- Carbohydrates: 35g
- Fat: 8g
- Fiber: 5g

Tips for Recipe Modification:

- Add sliced green onions for freshness.
- Use whole wheat noodles for added fiber.

MEDITERRANEAN QUINOA SALAD

Prep Time: 20 minutes

Ingredients (for one serving):

- 1/2 cup cooked quinoa
- 1/4 cup cherry tomatoes, halved
- 1/4 cup cucumber, diced
- 1/4 cup Kalamata olives, sliced
- Feta cheese for garnish
- Olive oil and lemon juice dressing

Cooking Instructions:

1. In a bowl, combine cooked quinoa, cherry tomatoes, diced cucumber, and sliced Kalamata olives.
2. Drizzle with olive oil and lemon juice dressing. Toss gently.
3. Garnish with crumbled feta cheese before serving.

Nutritional Information:

- Calories: 260
- Protein: 8g
- Carbohydrates: 35g
- Fat: 10g
- Fiber: 6g

Tips for Recipe Modification:

- Add diced red onion for extra flavor.
- Include chopped fresh parsley for a burst of freshness.

CAPRESE QUINOA SALAD

Prep Time: 15 minutes

Ingredients (for one serving):

- 1/2 cup cooked quinoa
- Cherry tomatoes, halved
- Fresh mozzarella balls
- Fresh basil leaves
- Balsamic glaze for dressing

Cooking Instructions:

1. In a bowl, combine cooked quinoa, cherry tomatoes, fresh mozzarella balls, and fresh basil leaves.
2. Drizzle with balsamic glaze. Toss gently.
3. Serve immediately.

Nutritional Information:

- Calories: 220
- Protein: 10g
- Carbohydrates: 25g
- Fat: 10g
- Fiber: 3g

Tips for Recipe Modification:

- Use whole-grain quinoa for added fiber.
- Drizzle with extra virgin olive oil for richness.

CHICKPEA AND AVOCADO SALAD

Prep Time: 15 minutes

Ingredients (for one serving):

- 1 cup canned chickpeas, rinsed and drained
- 1/2 avocado, diced
- 1/4 cup cherry tomatoes, halved
- Red onion, thinly sliced
- Cilantro, chopped
- Lime juice for dressing

Cooking Instructions:

1. In a bowl, combine chickpeas, diced avocado, cherry tomatoes, thinly sliced red onion, and chopped cilantro.
2. Drizzle with lime juice. Toss gently.
3. Serve chilled.

Nutritional Information:

- Calories: 280
- Protein: 10g
- Carbohydrates: 35g
- Fat: 14g
- Fiber: 10g

Tips for Recipe Modification:

- Add a pinch of cumin for a subtle smokiness.
- Include diced cucumber for extra crunch.

Prep Time: 15 minutes

Ingredients (for one serving):

- 4 ounces grilled chicken breast, sliced
- Mixed salad greens
- 1/2 apple, sliced
- 1/4 cup walnuts, chopped
- Blue cheese crumbles for garnish
- Apple cider vinaigrette for dressing

Cooking Instructions:

1. Arrange mixed salad greens on a plate.
2. Top with sliced grilled chicken, apple slices, chopped walnuts, and blue cheese crumbles.
3. Drizzle with apple cider vinaigrette. Serve chilled.

Nutritional Information:

- Calories: 320
- Protein: 25g
- Carbohydrates: 20g
- Fat: 18g
- Fiber: 5g

Tips for Recipe Modification:

- Use pecans or almonds for a different nutty flavor.
- Substitute blue cheese with feta for a milder taste.

Prep Time: 20 minutes

Ingredients (for one serving):

- 1/2 cup extra-firm tofu, cubed and stir-fried
- Mixed salad greens
- 1/4 cup bell peppers, sliced
- 1/4 cup snap peas, chopped
- 1/4 cup carrots, julienned
- Sesame soy dressing for flavor

Cooking Instructions:

1. Arrange mixed salad greens on a plate.
2. Top with stir-fried tofu, sliced bell peppers, chopped snap peas, and julienned carrots.
3. Drizzle with sesame soy dressing. Serve immediately.

Nutritional Information:

- Calories: 250
- Protein: 15g
- Carbohydrates: 25g
- Fat: 12g
- Fiber: 6g

Tips for Recipe Modification:

- Use tempeh as a plant-based protein alternative.
- Add a sprinkle of sesame seeds for extra crunch.

Prep Time: 15 minutes

Ingredients (for one serving):

- 4 ounces cooked shrimp
- Romaine lettuce, chopped
- 1/2 avocado, sliced
- 2 tablespoons Caesar dressing (low-sodium)
- 1 tablespoon grated Parmesan cheese

Cooking Instructions:

1. In a large bowl, combine chopped Romaine lettuce, cooked shrimp, and sliced avocado.
2. Drizzle with Caesar dressing and toss to coat evenly.
3. Sprinkle with grated Parmesan cheese before serving.

Nutritional Information:

- Calories: 280
- Protein: 25g
- Carbohydrates: 15g
- Fat: 15g
- Fiber: 5g

Tips for Recipe Modification:

- Use a whole-grain crouton for added texture.
- Substitute shrimp with grilled chicken if preferred.

MANGO AND BLACK BEAN QUINOA SALAD

Ingredients (for one serving):

- 1/2 cup cooked quinoa
- 1/2 cup black beans, canned and rinsed
- 1/4 cup mango, diced
- 1/4 cup red bell pepper, diced
- Fresh cilantro for garnish
- Lime vinaigrette for dressing

Cooking Instructions:

1. In a bowl, combine cooked quinoa, black beans, diced mango, and diced red bell pepper.
2. Drizzle with lime vinaigrette. Toss gently.
3. Garnish with fresh cilantro before serving.

Nutritional Information:

- Calories: 260
- Protein: 10g
- Carbohydrates: 40g
- Fat: 8g
- Fiber: 6g

Tips for Recipe Modification:

- Add a pinch of chili powder for a spicy kick.
- Include diced avocado for creaminess.

Prep Time: 15 minutes

Ingredients (for one serving):

- 1 can (5 oz.) tuna, drained
- 1/2 cup cannellini beans, canned and rinsed
- 1/4 cup red onion, finely chopped
- 1/4 cup cherry tomatoes, halved
- Kalamata olives for garnish
- Olive oil and red wine vinegar dressing

Cooking Instructions:

1. In a bowl, combine drained tuna, cannellini beans, finely chopped red onion, and halved cherry tomatoes.
2. Drizzle with olive oil and red wine vinegar dressing. Toss gently.
3. Garnish with Kalamata olives before serving.

Nutritional Information:

- Calories: 280
- Protein: 25g
- Carbohydrates: 25g
- Fat: 12g
- Fiber: 7g

Tips for Recipe Modification:

- Use tuna packed in olive oil for extra flavor.
- Add capers for a briny twist.

ROASTED BEET AND GOAT CHEESE SALAD

Prep Time: 25 minutes

Ingredients (for one serving):

- 1 medium beet, roasted and diced
- Mixed salad greens
- 1/4 cup goat cheese, crumbled
- Walnuts, chopped
- Balsamic glaze for dressing

Cooking Instructions:

1. Arrange mixed salad greens on a plate.
2. Top with roasted and diced beets, crumbled goat cheese, and chopped walnuts.
3. Drizzle with balsamic glaze. Serve chilled.

Nutritional Information:

- Calories: 250
- Protein: 8g
- Carbohydrates: 30g
- Fat: 14g
- Fiber: 6g

Tips for Recipe Modification:

- Use pecans or almonds for a different nutty flavor.
- Substitute goat cheese with feta for a milder taste.

SOUTHWEST CHICKEN SALAD

Prep Time: 20 minutes

Ingredients (for one serving):

- 4 ounces grilled chicken breast, sliced
- Romaine lettuce, chopped
- 1/4 cup corn kernels, fresh or frozen
- 1/4 cup black beans, canned and rinsed
- Avocado, sliced
- Salsa for dressing

Cooking Instructions:

1. In a large bowl, combine chopped Romaine lettuce, sliced grilled chicken, corn kernels, black beans, and sliced avocado.
2. Drizzle with salsa for a flavorful dressing. Toss gently.
3. Serve immediately.

Nutritional Information:

- Calories: 320
- Protein: 30g
- Carbohydrates: 20g
- Fat: 15g
- Fiber: 7g

Tips for Recipe Modification:

- Add a sprinkle of shredded cheddar cheese for extra richness.
- Use a lime-cilantro vinaigrette for a citrusy kick.

ORANGE AND FENNEL SALAD

Prep Time: 15 minutes

Ingredients (for one serving):

- Orange segments
- 1/4 cup fennel, thinly sliced
- Mixed salad greens
- 1/4 cup almonds, sliced
- Orange vinaigrette for dressing

Cooking Instructions:

- In a bowl, combine orange segments, thinly sliced fennel, mixed salad greens, and sliced almonds.
- Drizzle with orange vinaigrette. Toss gently.
- Serve chilled.

Nutritional Information:

- Calories: 220
- Protein: 6g
- Carbohydrates: 30g
- Fat: 10g
- Fiber: 7g

Tips for Recipe Modification:

- Add pomegranate seeds for a burst of color and flavor.
- Substitute almonds with pistachios for variety.

QUINOA AND ROASTED VEGETABLE SALAD

Prep Time: 30 minutes

Ingredients (for one serving):

- 1/2 cup cooked quinoa
- 1/2 cup cherry tomatoes, halved
- 1/4 cup bell peppers, diced
- 1/4 cup zucchini, sliced
- 1/4 cup red onion, thinly sliced
- Feta cheese for garnish
- Greek dressing for flavor

Cooking Instructions:

1. In a bowl, combine cooked quinoa, cherry tomatoes, diced bell peppers, sliced zucchini, and thinly sliced red onion.
2. Drizzle with Greek dressing. Toss gently.
3. Garnish with crumbled feta cheese before serving.

Nutritional Information:

- Calories: 280
- Protein: 8g
- Carbohydrates: 40g
- Fat: 10g
- Fiber: 6g

Tips for Recipe Modification:

- Add Kalamata olives for a Mediterranean touch.
- Grill the vegetables for a smoky flavor.

SEAFOOD RECIPES

BAKED LEMON GARLIC SALMON

Prep/Cook Time: 30 minutes

Ingredients (for one serving):

- 6 ounces salmon fillet
- 1 tablespoon olive oil
- 1 clove garlic, minced
- 1 tablespoon lemon juice
- Fresh dill for garnish

Cooking Instructions:

1. Preheat the oven to 375°F (190°C).
2. Place the salmon fillet on a baking sheet.
3. Mix olive oil, minced garlic, and lemon juice. Drizzle over the salmon.
4. Bake for 20-25 minutes until the salmon is cooked through.
5. Garnish with fresh dill before serving.

Nutritional Information:

- Calories: 300
- Protein: 30g
- Carbohydrates: 1g
- Fat: 20g
- Omega-3 Fatty Acids: 1.5g

- Add sliced cherry tomatoes for extra freshness.
- Use a lemon herb seasoning for added flavor.

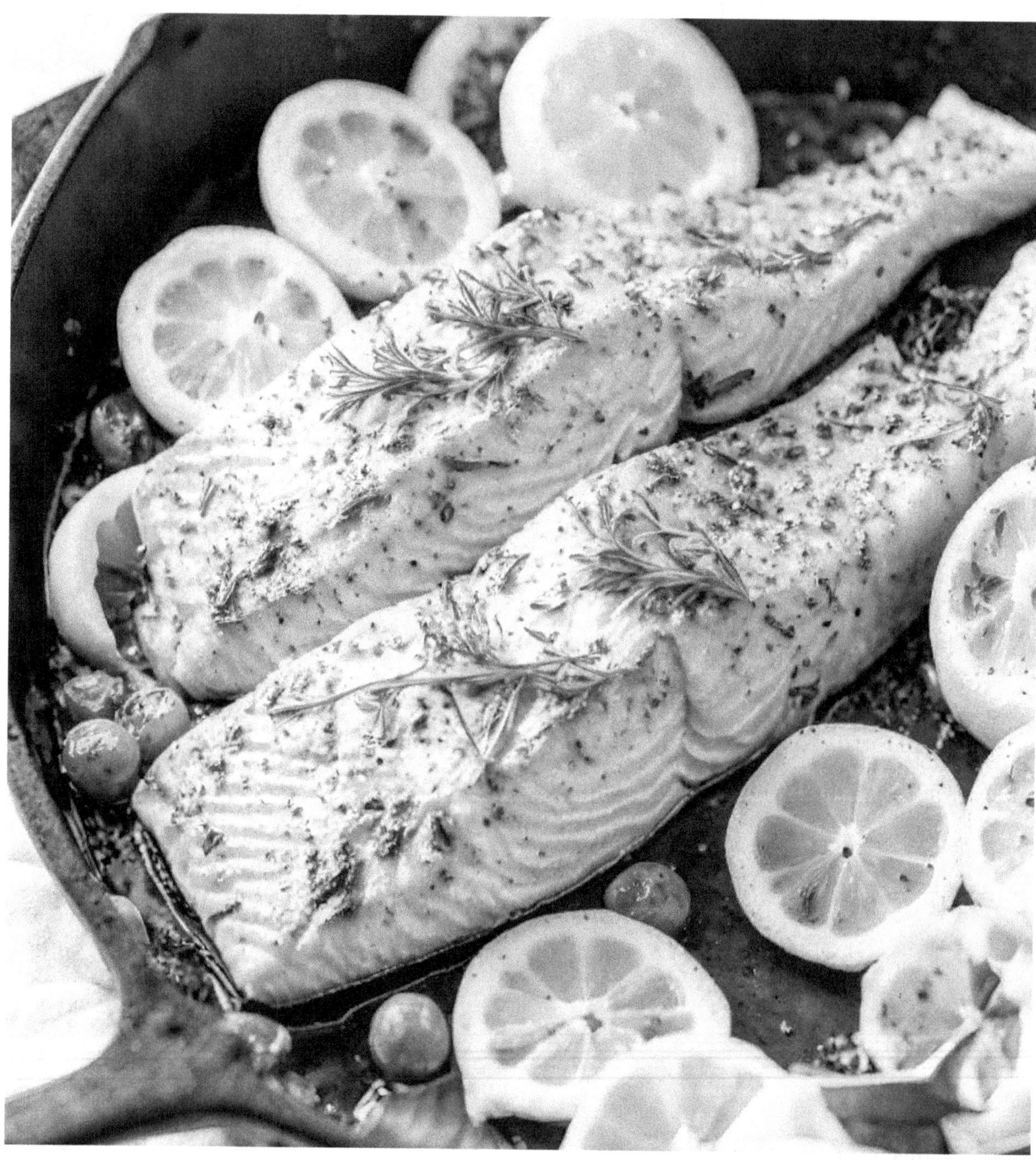

Prep/Cook Time: 20 minutes

Ingredients (for one serving):

- 8 large shrimp, peeled and deveined
- 1 tablespoon olive oil
- 1 teaspoon paprika
- 1/2 teaspoon garlic powder
- Fresh parsley for garnish

Cooking Instructions:

1. Preheat the grill or grill pan.
2. In a bowl, toss shrimp with olive oil, paprika, and garlic powder.
3. Thread shrimp onto skewers and grill for 2-3 minutes on each side.
4. Garnish with fresh parsley before serving.

Nutritional Information:

- Calories: 120
- Protein: 20g
- Carbohydrates: 1g
- Fat: 4g

Tips for Recipe Modification:

- Marinate shrimp in lemon juice for a citrusy twist.
- Add a pinch of cayenne pepper for a spicy kick.

BAKED TILAPIA WITH HERBS

Prep/Cook Time: 25 minutes

Ingredients (for one serving):

- 6 ounces tilapia fillet
- 1 tablespoon melted butter
- 1 teaspoon dried thyme
- 1 teaspoon dried rosemary
- Lemon wedges for serving

Cooking Instructions:

1. Preheat the oven to 400°F (200°C).
2. Place the tilapia fillet on a baking sheet.
3. Mix melted butter, dried thyme, and dried rosemary. Brush over the tilapia.
4. Bake for 15-18 minutes until the tilapia is cooked.
5. Serve with lemon wedges.

Nutritional Information:

- Calories: 200
- Protein: 25g
- Carbohydrates: 0g
- Fat: 11g

Tips for Recipe Modification:

- Use fresh herbs for a burst of flavor.
- Substitute butter with olive oil for a healthier option.

LEMON GARLIC BUTTER SCALLOPS

Prep/Cook Time: 15 minutes

Ingredients (for one serving):

- 8 large scallops
- 2 tablespoons unsalted butter
- 2 cloves garlic, minced
- 1 tablespoon lemon juice
- Chopped parsley for garnish

Cooking Instructions:

1. Pat scallops dry and season with salt and pepper.
2. In a skillet, melt butter over medium heat.
3. Add minced garlic and sauté for 1-2 minutes.
4. Add scallops and cook for 2-3 minutes on each side.
5. Drizzle with lemon juice and garnish with chopped parsley.

Nutritional Information:

- Calories: 180
- Protein: 20g
- Carbohydrates: 2g
- Fat: 10g

Tips for Recipe Modification:

- Use ghee for a lactose-free option.
- Add a splash of white wine for extra depth of flavor.

Prep/Cook Time: 25 minutes

Ingredients (for one serving):

- 6 ounces swordfish steak
- 1 tablespoon olive oil
- Zest of one lemon
- 1 teaspoon dried oregano
- Salt and pepper to taste

Cooking Instructions:

1. Preheat the grill or grill pan.
2. Brush swordfish with olive oil and sprinkle with lemon zest, dried oregano, salt, and pepper.
3. Grill for 4-5 minutes on each side or until cooked through.
4. Serve hot.

Nutritional Information:

- Calories: 250
- Protein: 30g
- Carbohydrates: 1g
- Fat: 14g

Tips for Recipe Modification:

- Replace dried oregano with fresh chopped parsley.
- Marinate swordfish in a lemon-garlic marinade for enhanced flavor.

HERB-ROASTED CHICKEN BREAST

Prep/Cook Time: 40 minutes

Ingredients (for one serving):

- 6 ounces chicken breast
- 1 tablespoon olive oil
- 1 teaspoon dried thyme
- 1 teaspoon dried rosemary
- Salt and pepper to taste

Cooking Instructions:

1. Preheat the oven to 375°F (190°C).
2. Rub chicken breast with olive oil, dried thyme, dried rosemary, salt, and pepper.
3. Place on a baking sheet and roast for 25-30 minutes or until cooked through.
4. Let it rest for a few minutes before slicing.

Nutritional Information:

- Calories: 280
- Protein: 30g
- Carbohydrates: 0g
- Fat: 16g

Tips for Recipe Modification:

- Add garlic powder for a savory kick.
- Use a meat thermometer to ensure proper cooking.

GRILLED LEMON HERB CHICKEN THIGHS

Prep/Cook Time: 30 minutes

Ingredients (for one serving):

- 2 chicken thighs, bone-in and skin-on
- 1 tablespoon olive oil
- Zest of one lemon
- 1 teaspoon dried oregano
- 1 teaspoon paprika
- Salt and pepper to taste

Cooking Instructions:

1. Preheat the grill or grill pan.
2. Mix olive oil, lemon zest, dried oregano, paprika, salt, and pepper.
3. Brush the mixture over chicken thighs and grill for 15-20 minutes, turning occasionally.
4. Ensure chicken reaches an internal temperature of 165°F (74°C).
5. Serve hot.

Nutritional Information:

- Calories: 320
- Protein: 25g
- Carbohydrates: 1g
- Fat: 22g

Tips for Recipe Modification:

- Add a squeeze of fresh lemon juice before serving.
- Marinate chicken thighs for a few hours for a more intense flavor.

.LEMON GARLIC TURKEY BURGERS

Prep/Cook Time: 20 minutes

Ingredients (for one serving):

- 6 ounces ground turkey
- 1 clove garlic, minced
- Zest of one lemon
- 1 tablespoon chopped fresh parsley
- Salt and pepper to taste
- Whole wheat burger bun

Cooking Instructions:

1. In a bowl, mix ground turkey, minced garlic, lemon zest, chopped parsley, salt, and pepper.
2. Form into a patty and grill for 8-10 minutes on each side or until fully cooked.
3. Toast the whole wheat burger bun and assemble the burger.
4. Serve with your choice of toppings.

Nutritional Information:

- Calories: 300
- Protein: 25g
- Carbohydrates: 20g
- Fat: 12g

Tips for Recipe Modification:

- Add a slice of tomato and lettuce for freshness.
- Use a low-sodium seasoning blend for reduced salt content.

BAKED HERB-CRUSTED CHICKEN DRUMSTICKS

Prep/Cook Time: 35 minutes

Ingredients (for one serving):

- 4 chicken drumsticks
- 1 tablespoon olive oil
- 1 teaspoon dried thyme
- 1 teaspoon dried rosemary
- 1/2 teaspoon garlic powder
- Salt and pepper to taste

Cooking Instructions:

1. Preheat the oven to 400°F (200°C).
2. Rub drumsticks with olive oil, dried thyme, dried rosemary, garlic powder, salt, and pepper.
3. Place on a baking sheet and bake for 25-30 minutes until the drumsticks are golden brown and cooked through.
4. Serve hot.

Nutritional Information:

- Calories: 250
- Protein: 25g
- Carbohydrates: 0g
- Fat: 16g

Tips for Recipe Modification:

- Use skinless drumsticks for a lower-fat option.
- Add a pinch of smoked paprika for a smoky flavor.

MEDITERRANEAN CHICKEN KABOBS

Prep/Cook Time: 30 minutes

Ingredients (for one serving):

- 6 ounces chicken breast, cut into cubes
- Cherry tomatoes
- Red onion, cut into chunks
- Bell peppers, cut into chunks
- Olive oil for brushing
- Greek seasoning for seasoning

Cooking Instructions:

1. Preheat the grill or grill pan.
2. Thread chicken cubes, cherry tomatoes, red onion, and bell peppers onto skewers.
3. Brush with olive oil and sprinkle with Greek seasoning.
4. Grill for 15-20 minutes, turning occasionally, until chicken is cooked.
5. Serve warm.

Nutritional Information:

- Calories: 300
- Protein: 30g
- Carbohydrates: 10g
- Fat: 14g

Tips for Recipe Modification:

- Marinate chicken in yogurt with garlic and herbs for added tenderness.
- Serve with a side of cucumber and mint tzatziki.

GARLIC PARMESAN BAKED COD

Prep/Cook Time: 20 minutes

Ingredients (for one serving):

- 6 ounces cod fillet
- 1 tablespoon melted butter
- 1 clove garlic, minced
- 2 tablespoons grated Parmesan cheese
- Fresh parsley for garnish

Cooking Instructions:

1. Preheat the oven to 400°F (200°C).
2. Place the cod fillet on a baking sheet.
3. Mix melted butter and minced garlic. Brush over the cod.
4. Sprinkle grated Parmesan cheese over the top.
5. Bake for 12-15 minutes until the cod is flaky.
6. Garnish with fresh parsley before serving.

Nutritional Information:

- Calories: 250
- Protein: 25g
- Carbohydrates: 1g
- Fat: 16g

Tips for Recipe Modification:

- Use olive oil instead of butter for a healthier option.
- Add a squeeze of lemon juice before serving.

BAKED DIJON MUSTARD CHICKEN THIGHS

Prep/Cook Time: 35 minutes

Ingredients (for one serving):

- 2 chicken thighs, bone-in and skin-on
- 1 tablespoon Dijon mustard
- 1 tablespoon olive oil
- 1 teaspoon dried thyme
- Salt and pepper to taste

Cooking Instructions:

1. Preheat the oven to 375°F (190°C).
2. Mix Dijon mustard, olive oil, dried thyme, salt, and pepper.
3. Rub the mixture over the chicken thighs and place them on a baking sheet.
4. Bake for 25-30 minutes until the chicken is cooked through.
5. Serve hot.

Nutritional Information:

- Calories: 320
- Protein: 25g
- Carbohydrates: 1g
- Fat: 22g

Tips for Recipe Modification:

- Add a sprinkle of smoked paprika for a smoky flavor.
- Use boneless, skinless chicken thighs for a leaner option.

LEMON ROSEMARY GRILLED CHICKEN BREAST

Prep/Cook Time: 30 *minutes*

Ingredients (for one serving):

- 6 ounces chicken breast
- 1 tablespoon olive oil
- Zest of one lemon
- 1 teaspoon dried rosemary
- Salt and pepper to taste

Cooking Instructions:

1. Preheat the grill or grill pan.
2. Brush chicken breast with olive oil and sprinkle with lemon zest, dried rosemary, salt, and pepper.
3. Grill for 15-20 minutes, turning occasionally, until chicken is cooked.
4. Let it rest for a few minutes before slicing.

Nutritional Information:

- Calories: 280
- Protein: 30g
- Carbohydrates: 0g
- Fat: 16g

Tips for Recipe Modification:

- Marinate chicken in the lemon-rosemary mixture for a few hours for enhanced flavor.
- Serve with a side of roasted vegetables.

SPINACH AND FETA STUFFED CHICKEN

Prep/Cook Time: 40 minutes

Ingredients (for one serving):

- 6 ounces chicken breast
- 1 cup fresh spinach, chopped
- 2 tablespoons feta cheese, crumbled
- 1 clove garlic, minced
- 1 teaspoon olive oil
- Salt and pepper to taste

Cooking Instructions:

1. Preheat the oven to 375°F (190°C).
2. In a skillet, sauté chopped spinach and minced garlic in olive oil until wilted.
3. Butterfly the chicken breast and stuff with sautéed spinach and feta cheese.
4. Bake for 25-30 minutes until the chicken is cooked.
5. Serve hot.

Nutritional Information:

- Calories: 320
- Protein: 30g
- Carbohydrates: 2g
- Fat: 20g

Tips for Recipe Modification:

- Add sun-dried tomatoes for a burst of sweetness.
- Use goat cheese as a flavorful alternative to feta.

CILANTRO LIME GRILLED CHICKEN THIGHS

Prep/Cook Time: 30 minutes

Ingredients (for one serving):

- 2 chicken thighs, bone-in and skin-on
- 2 tablespoons fresh cilantro, chopped
- Zest and juice of one lime
- 1 tablespoon olive oil
- Salt and pepper to taste

Cooking Instructions:

1. Preheat the grill or grill pan.
2. In a bowl, mix chopped cilantro, lime zest, lime juice, olive oil, salt, and pepper.
3. Brush the mixture over chicken thighs and grill for 15-20 minutes, turning occasionally.
4. Ensure chicken reaches an internal temperature of 165°F (74°C).
5. Serve hot.

Nutritional Information:

- Calories: 320
- Protein: 25g
- Carbohydrates: 2g
- Fat: 22g

Tips for Recipe Modification:

- Marinate chicken thighs for a few hours for a more intense flavor.
- Garnish with extra cilantro and lime wedges before serving.

BALSAMIC GLAZED CHICKEN DRUMSTICKS

Prep/Cook Time: 35 minutes

Ingredients (for one serving):

- 4 chicken drumsticks
- 2 tablespoons balsamic vinegar
- 1 tablespoon olive oil
- 1 teaspoon honey
- 1 teaspoon dried thyme
- Salt and pepper to taste

Cooking Instructions:

1. Preheat the oven to 400°F (200°C).
2. In a bowl, whisk together balsamic vinegar, olive oil, honey, dried thyme, salt, and pepper.
3. Rub drumsticks with the balsamic glaze and place on a baking sheet.
4. Bake for 25-30 minutes until the drumsticks are golden brown and cooked through.
5. Serve hot.

Nutritional Information:

- Calories: 280
- Protein: 25g
- Carbohydrates: 2g
- Fat: 18g

Tips for Recipe Modification:

- Add a pinch of garlic powder for extra flavor.
- Use a balsamic reduction for a thicker glaze.

MUSHROOM AND SWISS CHEESE STUFFED TURKEY BURGERS

Prep/Cook Time: 25 minutes

Ingredients (for one serving):

- 6 ounces ground turkey
- 1/4 cup mushrooms, finely chopped
- 2 tablespoons Swiss cheese, shredded
- 1 clove garlic, minced
- Salt and pepper to taste
- Whole wheat burger bun

Cooking Instructions:

1. In a bowl, mix ground turkey, chopped mushrooms, shredded Swiss cheese, minced garlic, salt, and pepper.
2. Form into a patty and grill for 8-10 minutes on each side or until fully cooked.
3. Toast the whole wheat burger bun and assemble the burger.
4. Serve with your choice of toppings.

Nutritional Information:

- Calories: 320
- Protein: 25g
- Carbohydrates: 20g
- Fat: 15g

Tips for Recipe Modification:

- Saute mushrooms with garlic before adding to the turkey mixture for enhanced flavor.
- Top the burger with sliced tomatoes and arugula.

DESSERT RECIPES

BERRY PARFAIT

Prep Time: 15 minutes

Ingredients (for one serving):

- 1/2 cup mixed berries (strawberries, blueberries, raspberries)
- 1/2 cup low-fat Greek yogurt
- 1 tablespoon honey
- 1 tablespoon chopped nuts (almonds or walnuts)

Cooking Instructions:

1. In a glass, layer mixed berries and Greek yogurt.
2. Drizzle honey over the top.
3. Sprinkle with chopped nuts for added crunch.

Nutritional Information:

- Calories: 150
- Protein: 8g
- Carbohydrates: 20g
- Fat: 6g
- Fiber: 4g

Tips for Recipe Modification:

- Use lactose-free yogurt for a dairy-free option.
- Add a sprinkle of cinnamon for extra flavor.

Prep Time: 5 minutes (+ overnight chilling)

Ingredients (for one serving):

- 2 tablespoons chia seeds
- 1/2 cup almond milk
- 1/2 teaspoon vanilla extract
- 1/2 cup diced mango

Cooking Instructions:

1. In a bowl, mix chia seeds, almond milk, and vanilla extract.
2. Refrigerate overnight or until the mixture thickens.
3. Top with diced mango before serving.

Nutritional Information:

- Calories: 180
- Protein: 5g
- Carbohydrates: 25g
- Fat: 8g
- Fiber: 8g

Tips for Recipe Modification:

- Experiment with different fruits like berries or kiwi.
- Add a touch of maple syrup for sweetness.

Prep/Cook Time: 30 minutes

Ingredients (for one serving):

- 1 medium apple, cored and sliced
- 1/2 teaspoon cinnamon
- 1 tablespoon chopped nuts (pecans or almonds)
- 1 teaspoon honey

Cooking Instructions:

1. Preheat the oven to 375°F (190°C).
2. Place apple slices in a baking dish and sprinkle with cinnamon.
3. Bake for 20-25 minutes until apples are tender.
4. Top with chopped nuts and drizzle with honey before serving.

Nutritional Information:

- Calories: 120
- Protein: 2g
- Carbohydrates: 20g
- Fat: 5g
- Fiber: 4g

Tips for Recipe Modification:

- Serve with a dollop of whipped cream for added indulgence.
- Add a pinch of nutmeg for a festive touch.

Prep/Cook Time: 45 minutes

Ingredients (for one serving):

- 1/4 cup Arborio rice
- 1 cup coconut milk
- 1/4 cup shredded coconut
- 1 tablespoon maple syrup
- 1/2 teaspoon vanilla extract

Cooking Instructions:

1. In a saucepan, combine Arborio rice, coconut milk, shredded coconut, maple syrup, and vanilla extract.
2. Simmer over low heat, stirring occasionally, until rice is cooked and mixture thickens.
3. Remove from heat and let it cool before serving.

Nutritional Information:

- Calories: 250
- Protein: 3g
- Carbohydrates: 30g
- Fat: 14g
- Fiber: 2g

Tips for Recipe Modification:

- Use unsweetened coconut milk for a lower sugar option.
- Top with fresh berries for a burst of color and flavor.

Prep Time: 10 minutes (+ freezing time)

Ingredients (for one serving):

- 1 banana, sliced
- 2 tablespoons peanut butter
- Dark chocolate chips for dipping

Instructions:

1. Spread peanut butter on banana slices and create banana sandwiches.
2. Dip each banana sandwich into melted dark chocolate chips.
3. Place on a tray and freeze until chocolate is set.

Nutritional Information:

- Calories: 180
- Protein: 4g
- Carbohydrates: 20g
- Fat: 10g
- Fiber: 3g

Tips for Recipe Modification:

- Use almond butter for a different nutty flavor.
- Sprinkle shredded coconut over the chocolate for variety.

CUCUMBER MINT INFUSED WATER

Prep Time: 5 minutes

Ingredients (for one serving):

- 1/2 cucumber, sliced
- Fresh mint leaves
- Ice cubes
- Water

Instructions:

1. In a pitcher, combine cucumber slices and fresh mint leaves.
2. Add ice cubes and fill the pitcher with water.
3. Let it infuse for at least 30 minutes before serving.

Tips for Recipe Modification:

- Add a splash of lemon juice for a citrusy twist.
- Use sparkling water for a fizzy variation.

HIBISCUS ICED TEA

Prep Time: 5 minutes (+ chilling time)

Ingredients (for one serving):

- 1 hibiscus tea bag
- 1 cup boiling water
- 1 tablespoon honey (optional)
- Ice cubes
- Lemon slices for garnish

Instructions:

1. Steep the hibiscus tea bag in boiling water for 5 minutes.
2. Add honey if desired and let it cool.
3. Refrigerate until chilled.
4. Serve over ice with lemon slices.

Tips for Recipe Modification:

- Experiment with other herbal teas like chamomile.
- Garnish with fresh berries for a burst of flavor.

Prep Time: 5 minutes

Ingredients (for one serving):

- 1/2 cup mixed berries (strawberries, blueberries, raspberries)
- 1/2 cup low-fat yogurt
- 1/2 cup almond milk
- 1 tablespoon chia seeds
- Ice cubes

Instructions:

1. In a blender, combine mixed berries, yogurt, almond milk, and chia seeds.
2. Blend until smooth.
3. Add ice cubes and blend again until well combined.

Nutritional Information:

- Calories: 150
- Protein: 6g
- Carbohydrates: 20g
- Fat: 5g
- Fiber: 5g

Tips for Recipe Modification:

- Use frozen berries for a colder and thicker consistency.
- Add a banana for extra creaminess.

TURMERIC GOLDEN MILK

Prep/Cook Time: 10 minutes

Ingredients (for one serving):

- 1 cup unsweetened almond milk
- 1/2 teaspoon ground turmeric
- 1/4 teaspoon ground cinnamon
- 1/4 teaspoon ground ginger
- 1 tablespoon honey (optional)

Instructions:

1. In a saucepan, heat almond milk over medium heat.
2. Whisk in turmeric, cinnamon, and ginger.
3. Stir until well combined and heated through.
4. Sweeten with honey if desired.

Nutritional Information:

- Calories: 80
- Protein: 2g
- Carbohydrates: 10g
- Fat: 3g
- Fiber: 1g

Tips for Recipe Modification:

- Use coconut milk for a different flavor.
- Add a pinch of black pepper to enhance turmeric absorption.

AVOCADO AND SPINACH SMOOTHIE

Prep Time: 5 minutes

Ingredients (for one serving):

- 1/2 ripe avocado
- 1 cup fresh spinach
- 1/2 banana
- 1/2 cup almond milk
- Ice cubes

Instructions:

1. In a blender, combine ripe avocado, fresh spinach, banana, and almond milk.
2. Blend until smooth.
3. Add ice cubes and blend again until well combined.

Nutritional Information:

- Calories: 200
- Protein: 4g
- Carbohydrates: 20g
- Fat: 12g
- Fiber: 7g

Tips for Recipe Modification:

- Add a scoop of protein powder for an extra protein boost.
- Squeeze in a bit of lime juice for brightness.

MINT CHOCOLATE CHIP SMOOTHIE

Prep Time: 5 minutes

Ingredients (for one serving):

- 1/2 cup fresh mint leaves
- 1/2 banana
- 1 cup almond milk
- 1 tablespoon dark chocolate chips
- Ice cubes

Instructions:

1. In a blender, combine fresh mint leaves, banana, almond milk, and dark chocolate chips.
2. Blend until smooth.
3. Add ice cubes and blend again until well combined.

Nutritional Information:

- Calories: 180
- Protein: 4g
- Carbohydrates: 25g
- Fat: 8g
- Fiber: 5g

Tips for Recipe Modification:

- Use cacao nibs for a richer chocolate flavor.
- Garnish with a sprig of mint for presentation.

Prep Time: 5 minutes

Ingredients (for one serving):

- 1/2 cup pineapple chunks
- 1/2 teaspoon grated ginger
- Sparkling water
- Ice cubes
- Fresh mint for garnish

Instructions:

1. In a glass, muddle pineapple chunks and grated ginger.
2. Fill the glass with ice cubes.
3. Pour sparkling water over the mixture.
4. Garnish with fresh mint before serving.

Tips for Recipe Modification:

- Use frozen pineapple chunks for a colder beverage.
- Add a splash of coconut water for a tropical twist.

CRANBERRY LIME MOCKTAIL

Prep Time: 5 minutes

Ingredients (for one serving):

- 1/2 cup cranberry juice (unsweetened)
- Juice of one lime
- Soda water
- Ice cubes
- Lime slices for garnish

Instructions:

1. In a glass, combine cranberry juice and lime juice.
2. Fill the glass with ice cubes.
3. Top with soda water and stir gently.
4. Garnish with lime slices before serving.

Tips for Recipe Modification:

- Use a cranberry-lime flavored seltzer for added fizz.
- Sweeten with a bit of honey if desired.

MANGO MINT GREEN TEA

Prep/Cook Time: 10 minutes

Ingredients (for one serving):

- 1 green tea bag
- 1 cup boiling water
- 1/2 cup diced mango
- Fresh mint leaves
- Ice cubes

Instructions:

1. Steep the green tea bag in boiling water for 3-5 minutes.
2. Let the tea cool to room temperature.
3. In a glass, combine diced mango and fresh mint leaves.
4. Pour the cooled green tea over the mango and mint.
5. Add ice cubes before serving.

Tips for Recipe Modification:

- Use honey or agave syrup to sweeten the tea.
- Garnish with a slice of lime for a citrusy touch.

PEACH BASIL LEMONADE

Prep/Cook Time: 15 minutes

Ingredients (for one serving):

- 1/2 cup fresh peach slices
- 2-3 fresh basil leaves
- Juice of one lemon
- 1 tablespoon honey
- Still or sparkling water
- Ice cubes

Instructions:

1. In a blender, blend fresh peach slices, basil leaves, lemon juice, and honey until smooth.
2. Strain the mixture to remove pulp.
3. In a glass, combine the strained peach-basil-lemon mixture with still or sparkling water.
4. Add ice cubes before serving.

Tips for Recipe Modification:

- Replace basil with mint for a different herbaceous flavor.
- Adjust honey according to sweetness preference.

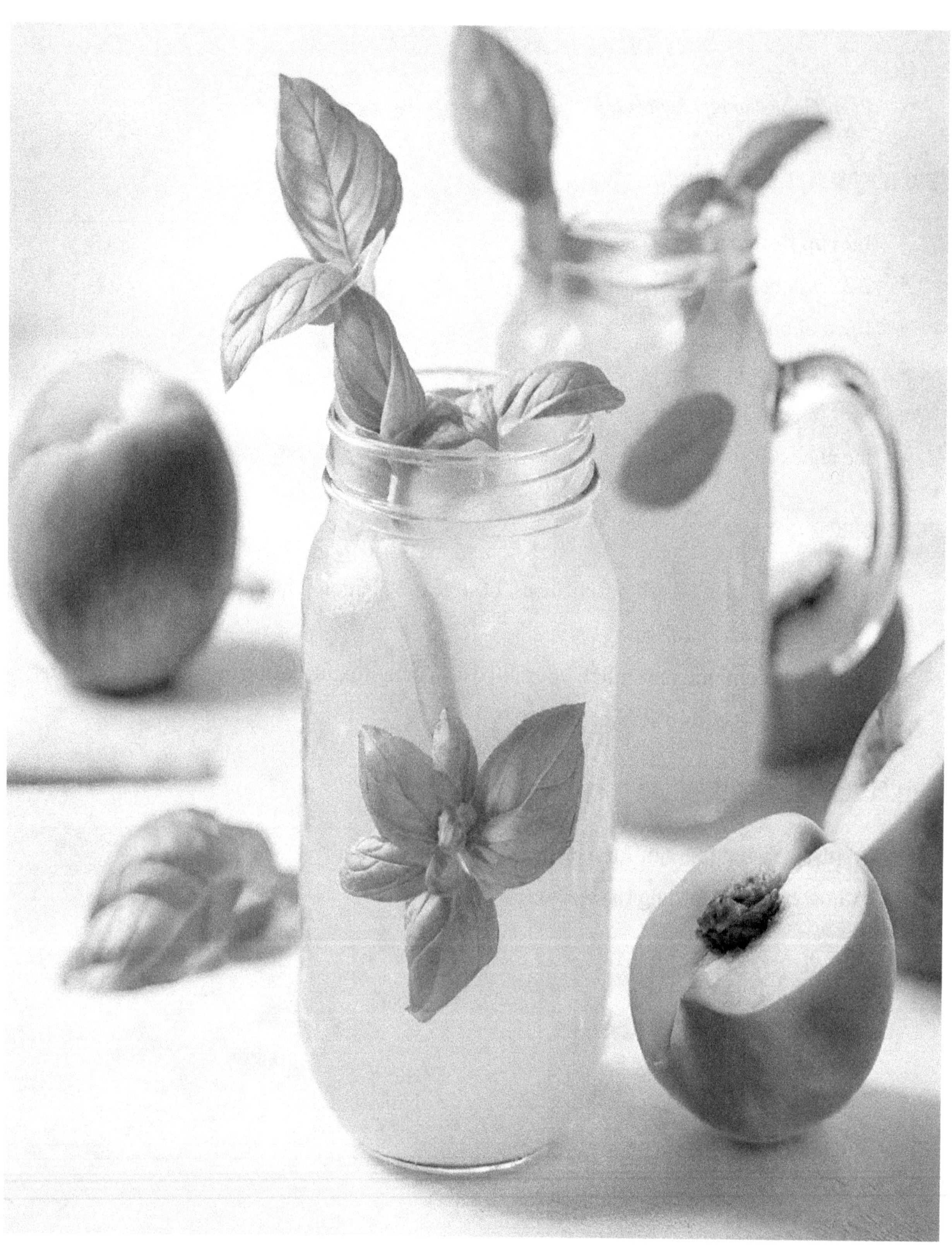

DAY	BREAKFAST	LUNCH	DINNER	SNACK
WEEK 1				
Monday	Vegetable Omelette	Grilled Lemon Herb Chicken	Baked Lemon Herb Tilapia	Hummus and Veggie Sticks
Tuesday	Quinoa Breakfast Bowl	Quinoa Salad with Vegetables	Cauliflower Rice and Turkey Stuffed Peppers	Cucumber and Tuna Bites
Wednesday	Sweet Potato Hash	Baked Salmon with Asparagus	Salmon and Asparagus Foil Packets	Avocado and Tomato Salsa
Thursday	Greek Yogurt Parfait	Mediterranean Chickpea Salad	Vegetarian Eggplant Lasagna	Egg Salad Lettuce Wraps
Friday	Cottage Cheese Pancakes	Turkey and Avocado Wrap	Grilled Chicken and Quinoa Salad	Baked Parmesan Zucchini Chips
Saturday	Egg and Spinach Breakfast Wrap	Eggplant and Tomato Stew	Lemon Garlic Shrimp and Broccoli Stir-Fry	Peanut Butter Banana Bites
Sunday	Chia Seed Pudding	Lemon Garlic Shrimp Stir-Fry	Quinoa and Black Bean Stuffed Bell Peppers	Cottage Cheese and Pineapple Bowl
WEEK 2				
Monday	Mushroom and Spinach Frittata	Vegetarian Lentil Soup	Turkey and Vegetable Skewers with Yogurt Sauce	Cherry Almond Energy Bites

Tuesday	Almond Flour Pancakes	Chicken and Vegetable Skewers	Vegetable and Tofu Stir-Fry with Brown Rice	Smoked Salmon Cucumber Rolls
Wednesday	Tomato and Basil Egg Muffins	Stuffed Bell Peppers with Turkey	Mushroom and Spinach Risotto	Stuffed Cherry Tomatoes with Tuna
Thursday	Peanut Butter Banana Smoothie	Egg Fried Rice with Vegetables	Chicken and Broccoli Quinoa Bowl	Baked Apple Chips
Friday	Spinach and Tomato Breakfast Wrap	Shrimp and Broccoli Alfredo	Vegetarian Lentil and Vegetable Curry	Spicy Edamame
Saturday	Blueberry Almond Muffins	Cauliflower and Chickpea Curry	Mediterranean Grilled Vegetable Skewers	Quinoa and Cranberry Stuffed Dates
Sunday	Cinnamon Raisin Overnight Oats	Spinach and Feta Stuffed Chicken Breast	Shrimp and Vegetable Stir-Fry with Brown Rice	Caprese Salad Skewers
WEEK 3				
Monday	Salmon and Avocado Toast	Caprese Salad with Balsamic Glaze	Lemon Herb Baked Chicken Thighs	Walnut and Berry Salad
Tuesday	Vegetable Omelette	Pesto Zoodles with Cherry Tomatoes	Cabbage and Chicken Sauté	Cinnamon Roasted Almonds
Wednesday	Quinoa Breakfast Bowl	Mediterranean Grilled Vegetable Skewers	Stuffed Portobello Mushrooms with Turkey	Mango Salsa with Baked Pita Chips

Day				
Thursday	Sweet Potato Hash	Shrimp and Vegetable Stir-Fry with Brown Rice	Mediterranean Shrimp and Quinoa Bowl	Chia Seed Pudding with Berries
Friday	Greek Yogurt Parfait	Tomato Basil Grilled Chicken	Baked Dijon Mustard Chicken Thighs	Cucumber and Greek Yogurt Dip
Saturday	Cottage Cheese Pancakes	Lemon Rosemary Grilled Chicken Breast	Mushroom and Swiss Cheese Stuffed Turkey Burgers	Pumpkin Seed Trail Mix
Sunday	Egg and Spinach Breakfast Wrap	Vegetarian Zucchini Lasagna	Grilled Lemon Herb Chicken Thighs	Sun-Dried Tomato and Basil Rice Cakes

WEEK 4

Day				
Monday	Blueberry Almond Muffins	Spinach and Feta Stuffed Chicken Breast	Shrimp and Vegetable Stir-Fry with Brown Rice	Caprese Salad Skewers
Tuesday	Cinnamon Raisin Overnight Oats	Cauliflower and Chickpea Curry	Mediterranean Grilled Vegetable Skewers	Quinoa and Cranberry Stuffed Dates
Wednesday	Salmon and Avocado Toast	Caprese Salad with Balsamic Glaze	Lemon Herb Baked Chicken Thighs	Walnut and Berry Salad
Thursday	Vegetable Omelette	Pesto Zoodles with Cherry Tomatoes	Cabbage and Chicken Sauté	Cinnamon Roasted Almonds
Friday	Quinoa Breakfast Bowl	Mediterranean Grilled Vegetable Skewers	Stuffed Portobello Mushrooms with Turkey	Mango Salsa with Baked Pita Chips

Saturday	Sweet Potato Hash	Shrimp and Vegetable Stir-Fry with Brown Rice	Mediterranean Shrimp and Quinoa Bowl	Chia Seed Pudding with Berries
Sunday	Cottage Cheese Pancakes	Lemon Rosemary Grilled Chicken Breast	Mushroom and Swiss Cheese Stuffed Turkey Burgers	Cucumber and Greek Yogurt Dip

NOTE:

Feel free to mix and match the meals, and adjust portion sizes based on individual dietary needs and remember to stay hydrated.

GROCERY SHOPPING LIST FOR A KIDNEY-FRIENDLY DIET

1. PROTEINS	<ul><li>Chicken breasts</li><li>Turkey (ground, breast)</li><li>Salmon fillets</li><li>Tilapia fillets</li><li>Shrimp</li><li>Eggs</li><li>Tofu</li><li>Cottage cheese</li><li>Greek yogurt</li><li>Canned tuna (in water)</li></ul>
2. GRAINS	<ul><li>Quinoa</li><li>Brown rice</li><li>Arborio rice</li><li>Barley</li><li>Whole wheat flour</li></ul>

	• Almond flour
3. VEGETABLES	• Spinach • Kale • Eggplant • Bell peppers (variety of colors) • Mushrooms • Zucchini • Tomatoes • Sweet potatoes • Cauliflower • Asparagus • Broccoli • Cabbage • Avocado • Portobello mushrooms • Fennel • Garlic • Onion
4. FRUITS	• Berries (strawberries, blueberries, raspberries) • Bananas • Apples • Mango • Lemon • Lime • Orange • Peach • Watermelon

5. LEGUMES	<ul><li>Chickpeas</li><li>Lentils</li><li>Black beans</li><li>White beans</li></ul>
6. DAIRY AND DAIRY ALTERNATIVES	<ul><li>Low-fat cheese (Swiss, feta)</li><li>Almond milk (unsweetened)</li><li>Coconut milk (unsweetened)</li><li>Yogurt (low-fat, plain or Greek)</li><li>Parmesan cheese</li></ul>
7. NUTS AND SEEDS	<ul><li>Almonds</li><li>Walnuts</li><li>Pecans</li><li>Chia seeds</li><li>Pumpkin seeds</li></ul>
8. HERBS AND SPICES	<ul><li>Basil</li><li>Cilantro</li><li>Dill</li><li>Mint</li><li>Oregano</li><li>Parsley</li><li>Rosemary</li><li>Thyme</li><li>Garlic powder</li><li>Onion powder</li><li>Turmeric</li><li>Cinnamon</li><li>Paprika</li></ul>

	• Dijon mustard
9. OILS AND VINEGARS	• Olive oil • Avocado oil • Balsamic vinegar • Apple cider vinegar
10. CONDIMENTS AND SAUCES	• Hummus • Salsa • Pesto • Dijon mustard • Soy sauce (low sodium) • Fish sauce • Lemon juice • Honey (for those without restrictions) • Coconut aminos
11. CANNED GOODS	• Low-sodium chicken or vegetable broth • Diced tomatoes (no added salt) • Tomato paste • Coconut milk (unsweetened)
12. FROZEN FOODS	• Frozen berries • Frozen shrimp • Frozen vegetables (mixed)
13. BAKERY	• Brown rice cakes • Whole wheat pita bread
14. MISCELLANEOUS	• Edamame (shelled) • Quinoa flakes

	• Unsweetened coconut flakes • Dark chocolate chips (for moderation)
15. BEVERAGES	• Water • Herbal tea bags (hibiscus, chamomile) • Sparkling water
16. SWEETENERS	• Stevia (for those without restrictions) • Agave syrup (in moderation, for those without restrictions)

PHYSICAL ACTIVITIES TO SUPPORT CKD MANAGEMENT

7-DAY EXERCISE PLAN

Day 1: Cardiovascular Exercise

- **Activity:** Brisk walking
- **Duration:** 30 minutes
- **Intensity:** Moderate

Notes: Focus on maintaining a steady pace. Use a pedometer or fitness tracker to monitor steps.

Day 2: Strength Training

- **Activity:** Bodyweight exercises (e.g., squats, lunges, push-ups)
- **Duration:** 20 minutes
- **Intensity:** Light to moderate

Notes: Perform each exercise with proper form. Start with a set of 10-15 repetitions.

Day 3: Flexibility and Balance

- **Activity:** Yoga or Tai Chi
- **Duration:** 20 minutes
- **Intensity:** Low to moderate

Notes: Emphasize gentle stretching and balance poses. Follow an instructional video if needed.

Day 4: Cardiovascular Exercise

- **Activity:** Stationary cycling or swimming
- **Duration:** 30 minutes
- **Intensity:** Moderate

Notes: Choose a low-impact option. Swimming is gentle on the joints.

Day 5: Rest or Light Activity

- **Activity:** Gentle stretching or a short walk
- **Duration:** 15-20 minutes
- **Intensity:** Low

Notes: Allow your body to recover with light activity. Focus on deep breathing.

Day 6: Strength Training

- **Activity:** Resistance band exercises or light dumbbell workouts
- **Duration:** 20 minutes
- **Intensity:** Light to moderate

Notes: Perform controlled movements to target different muscle groups.

Day 7: Cardiovascular Exercise and Relaxation

- **Activity:** Walking or easy cycling
- **Duration:** 30 minutes
- **Intensity:** Light

Notes: Enjoy a leisurely walk or bike ride. Include deep breathing exercises for relaxation.

Additional Tips:

1. **Hydration:** Drink water before, during, and after exercise to stay well-hydrated.
2. **Warm-up:** Prioritize a 5-10 minute warm-up before each session to prepare your muscles.
3. **Cool-down:** Finish each session with a 5-10 minute cool-down, including stretching.
4. **Listen to your body:** If you experience pain or discomfort, modify or stop the activity. Consult your healthcare provider if needed.
5. **Consistency is key:** Aim for at least 150 minutes of moderate-intensity exercise per week, as recommended by health guidelines.

Always tailor the exercise plan to your fitness level and medical condition. If you have specific concerns or conditions related to CKD, consult me via consultemilywilson@gmail.com for a personalized advice.

CONCLUSION

In the journey toward better health and well-being, the understanding of Chronic Kidney Disease (CKD) is not merely a matter of medical terminology; it is a compass guiding us towards informed decisions that impact our daily lives. As we navigated through Chapter One of this CKD Diet Cookbook, we delved into the intricacies of CKD – unraveling its stages, identifying its common causes, and acknowledging the vital role our kidneys play in maintaining our overall health.

In Chapter Two, we explored the empowering realm of managing CKD through conscious choices in our diet and lifestyle. The knowledge shared about dietary guidelines, renal-friendly foods, and nutrient-rich options is not just information; it's a tool for transforming our daily meals into nourishing support for our kidneys. By understanding foods to embrace and those to avoid, we embark on a culinary journey that goes beyond taste; it becomes a commitment to kidney health.

The heart of this cookbook lies in the diverse array of recipes meticulously crafted for those managing CKD. From delightful breakfast options to satisfying dinners, every recipe is a celebration of flavors tailored to suit the needs of your kidneys. The 30-day meal plan provides structure and variety, ensuring that your journey towards better kidney health is both enjoyable and sustainable.

As we advocate for the well-being of our kidneys, we acknowledge that a holistic approach extends beyond the kitchen. The 7-day exercise plan included is not just a series of physical activities; it's a guide to embracing an active lifestyle that complements your dietary efforts. By combining nutritious recipes with purposeful physical activity, you are laying the foundation for a healthier, more vibrant life.

In conclusion, this CKD Diet Cookbook is more than a collection of recipes; it is a roadmap for transforming the way you nourish your body and support your kidneys. Each page is infused with the dedication to empower you on your journey towards managing CKD. Remember, you are not alone on this path – your choices matter, and they contribute to the well-being of your kidneys.

Here's to your health, your journey, and the power within you to make a difference, one delicious and kidney-friendly choice at a time.

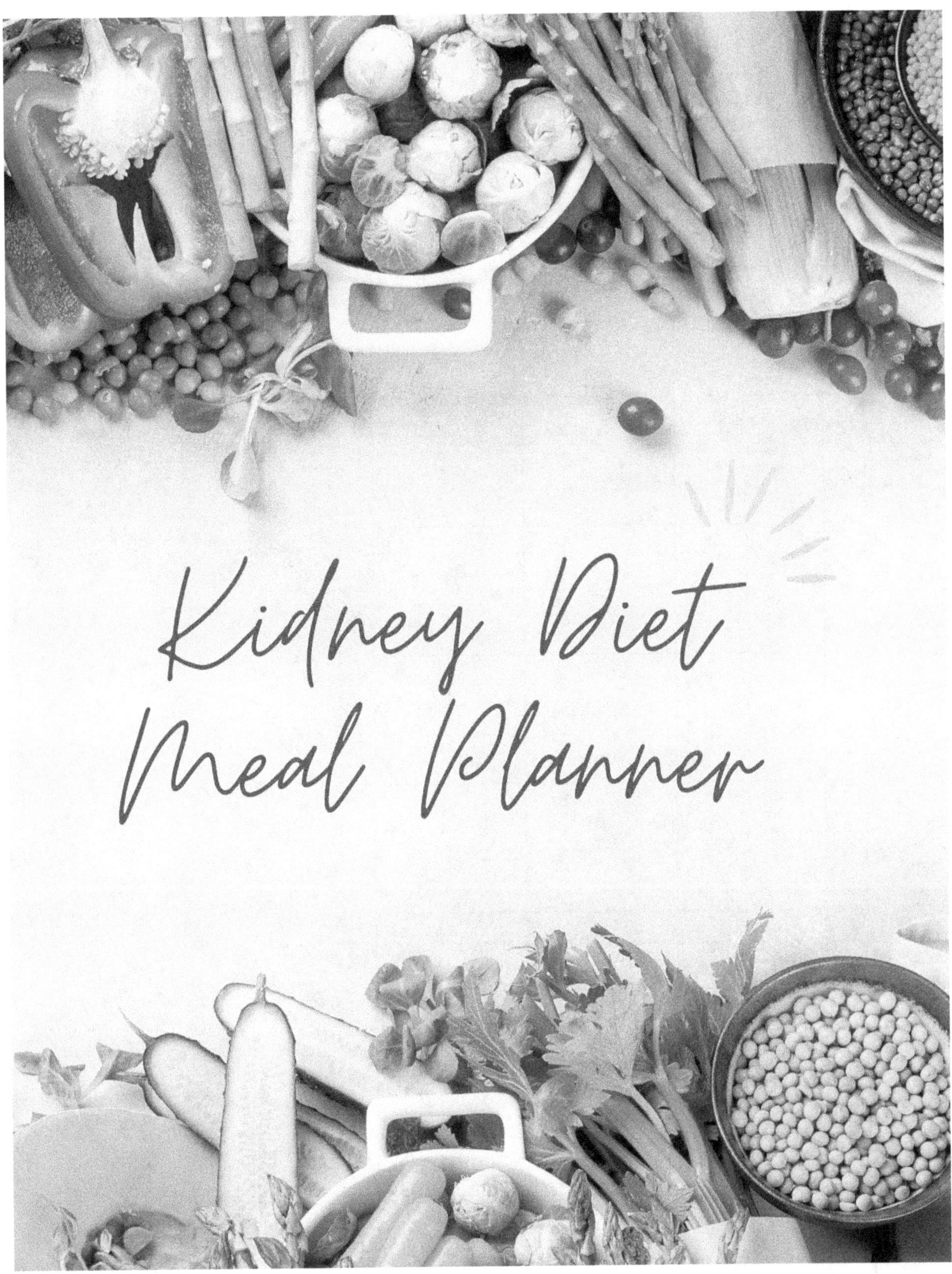

Kidney Diet Meal Planner

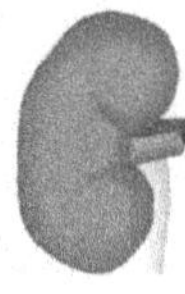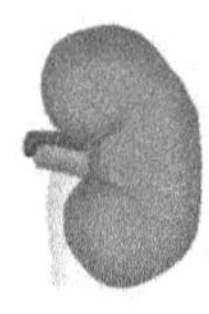

KIDNEY DIET
Meal Planner

	BREAKFAST	LUNCH	DINNER
MON			
TUE			
WED			
THU			
FRI			
SAT			
SUN			

Your strength shines brightest in the face of adversity.
Keep shining; you are a beacon of hope

Date:
....

Shopping List

Note:

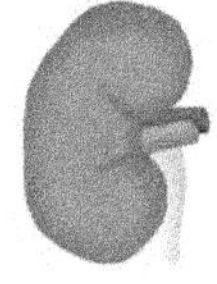 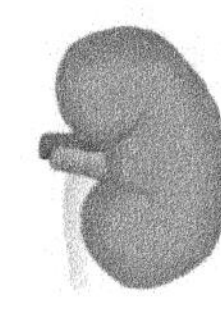# KIDNEY DIET
Meal Planner

Date:

Shopping List

	BREAKFAST	LUNCH	DINNER
MON			
TUE			
WED			
THU			
FRI			
SAT			
SUN			

Your health is a reflection of the choices you make every day. Choose wisely, and you'll create a brighter future.

Note:

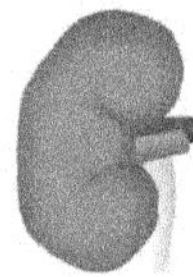# KIDNEY DIET
Meal Planner

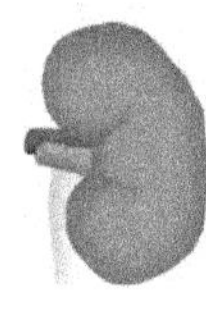

Date:
....

Shopping List

	BREAKFAST	LUNCH	DINNER
MON			
TUE			
WED			
THU			
FRI			
SAT			
SUN			

The path to healing begins with self-compassion. Be kind to yourself as you navigate this journey

Note:

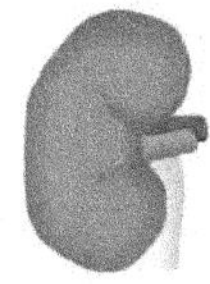 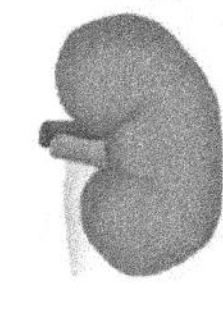

KIDNEY DIET
Meal Planner

	BREAKFAST	LUNCH	DINNER
MON			
TUE			
WED			
THU			
FRI			
SAT			
SUN			

Patience is your greatest ally. Healing takes time, but every day brings you closer to your goals.

Date:
....

Shopping List

Note:

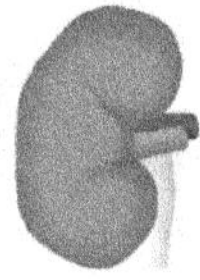 # KIDNEY DIET
Meal Planner
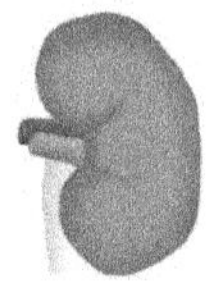

	BREAKFAST	LUNCH	DINNER
MON			
TUE			
WED			
THU			
FRI			
SAT			
SUN			

Surround yourself with positivity and people who believe in your ability to overcome. Together, you are unstoppable

Date:
....

Shopping List

Note:

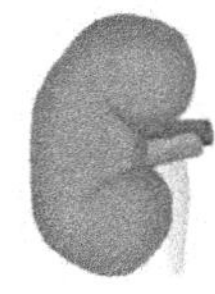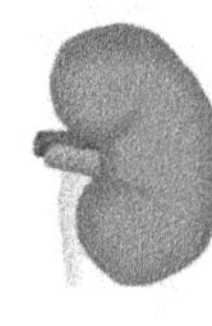

KIDNEY DIET
Meal Planner

	BREAKFAST	LUNCH	DINNER
MON			
TUE			
WED			
THU			
FRI			
SAT			
SUN			

The journey to wellness may be long, but remember, you have the strength to make it.

Date:
....

Shopping List

Note:

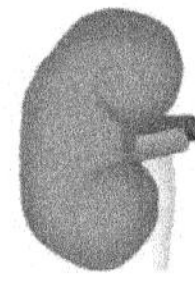# KIDNEY DIET
Meal Planner

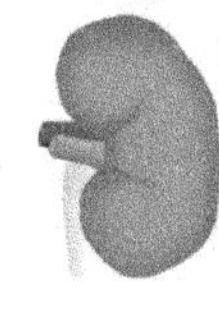

	BREAKFAST	LUNCH	DINNER
MON			
TUE			
WED			
THU			
FRI			
SAT			
SUN			

Hope is the heartbeat of resilience. Keep it alive, and you can conquer any obstacle.

Date:
....

Shopping List

Note:

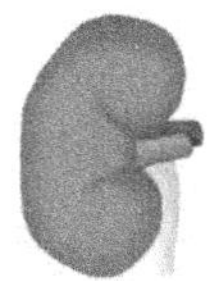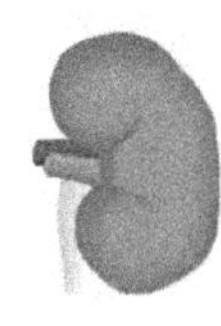

KIDNEY DIET
Meal Planner

	BREAKFAST	LUNCH	DINNER
MON			
TUE			
WED			
THU			
FRI			
SAT			
SUN			

Your body is an incredible masterpiece. It has the power to heal and recover with the right care and love.

Date:
....

Shopping List

Note:

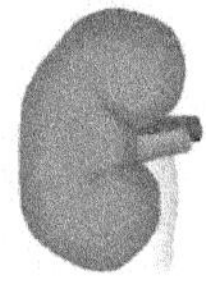 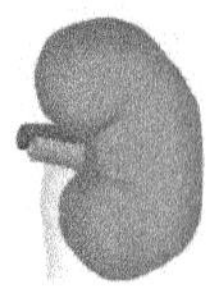

KIDNEY DIET
Meal Planner

Date:
....

Shopping List

	BREAKFAST	LUNCH	DINNER
MON			
TUE			
WED			
THU			
FRI			
SAT			
SUN			

You are not defined by your diagnosis; you are defined by your courage and determination

Note:

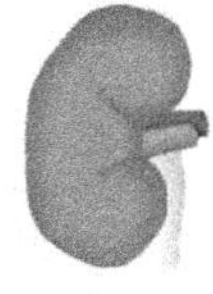 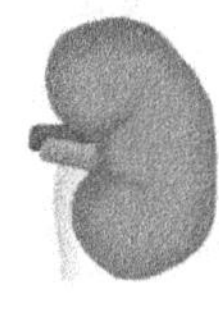

KIDNEY DIET
Meal Planner

	BREAKFAST	LUNCH	DINNER
MON			
TUE			
WED			
THU			
FRI			
SAT			
SUN			

Small steps can lead to significant changes. Each healthy choice you make brings you closer to wellness.

Date:
....

Shopping List

Note:

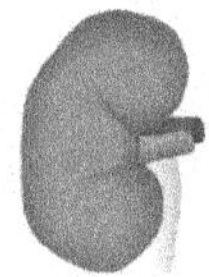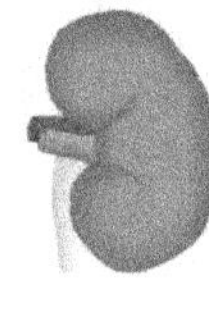

KIDNEY DIET
Meal Planner

	BREAKFAST	LUNCH	DINNER
MON			
TUE			
WED			
THU			
FRI			
SAT			
SUN			

You are stronger than you know, and your spirit is more resilient than any challenge. Keep fighting, and never lose hope.

Date:
....

Shopping List

Note:

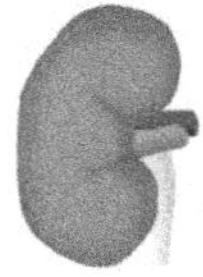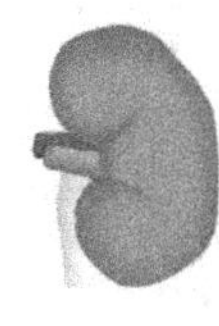

KIDNEY DIET
Meal Planner

	BREAKFAST	LUNCH	DINNER
MON			
TUE			
WED			
THU			
FRI			
SAT			
SUN			

Date:
....

Shopping List

Note:

In the journey of life, challenges like kidney disease are just detours. Keep moving forward; your destination is worth the fight

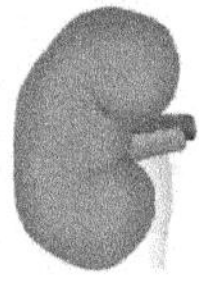# KIDNEY DIET
Meal Planner

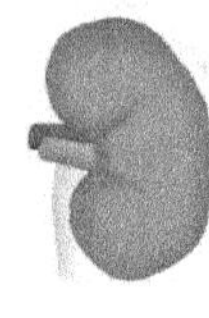

Date:
....

Shopping List

	BREAKFAST	LUNCH	DINNER
MON			
TUE			
WED			
THU			
FRI			
SAT			
SUN			

Your health is your most precious asset. Treat it with love, care, and the right nutrition.

Note:

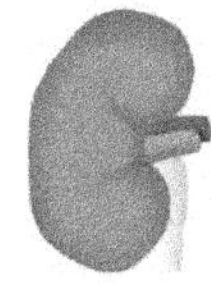 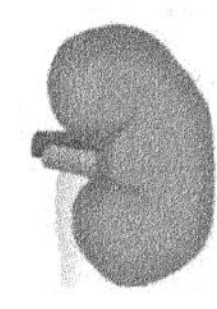

KIDNEY DIET
Meal Planner

	BREAKFAST	LUNCH	DINNER
MON			
TUE			
WED			
THU			
FRI			
SAT			
SUN			

Believe in your inner strength; it's the fuel that keeps you going even when the road gets tough.

Date:

....

Shopping List

Note:

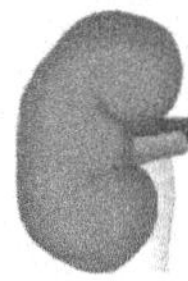 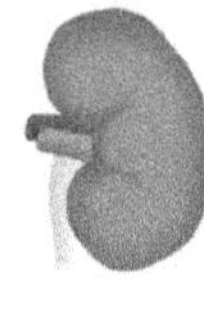

KIDNEY DIET
Meal Planner

	BREAKFAST	LUNCH	DINNER
MON			
TUE			
WED			
THU			
FRI			
SAT			
SUN			

Every meal is a chance to nourish your body and nurture your kidneys. Embrace each bite as a step towards better health.

Date:
....

Shopping List

Note:

www.ingramcontent.com/pod-product-compliance
Lightning Source LLC
Chambersburg PA
CBHW080845260726
48660CB00009B/3208